# FIFTEEN YEARS
# IN HELL

## AN AUTOBIOGRAPHY

## LUTHER BENSON

# Fifteen Years in Hell

## Luther Benson

© 1st World Library – Literary Society, 2006
PO Box 2211
Fairfield, IA 52556
www.1stworldlibrary.org
First Edition

LCCN: 2006930797

Softcover ISBN: 1-4218-2197-4
Hardcover ISBN: 1-4218-2097-8
eBook ISBN: 1-4218-2297-0

Purchase *"Fifteen Years in Hell"*
as a traditional bound book at:
www.1stWorldLibrary.org/purchase.asp?ISBN=1-4218-2197-4

1st World Library Literary Society is a nonprofit
organization dedicated to promoting literacy by:

- Creating a free internet library accessible from any
  computer worldwide.
- Hosting writing competitions and offering book
  publishing scholarships.

Readers interested in supporting literacy
through sponsorship, donations or
membership please contact:
literacy@1stworldlibrary.org
Check us out at: www.1stworldlibrary.ORG
and start downloading free ebooks today.

***Fifteen Years in Hell***
*contributed by Tim, Ed & Rodney*
*in support of*
*1st World Library Literary Society*

# TABLE OF CONTENTS

My parents' shame and sorrow - My own remorse -
An unhappy and silent breakfast - The anguish of
my mother - Gradual recovery - Resolves and
promises - No pleasure in drinking - The system's
final craving for liquor - The hopelessness of the
drunkard's condition - The resistless power of
appetite - Possible escape - The courage required -
The three laws - Their violation and man's
atonement.

School days at Fairview - My first public outbreak -
A schoolmate - Drive to Falmouth - First drink at
Falmouth - Disappointment - Drive to Smelser's
Mills - Hostetter's Bitters - The author's opinion of
patent medicines, bitters especially - Boasting -
More liquor - Difficulty in lighting a cigar - A
hound that got in bad company - Oysters at
Falmouth, and what befell us while waiting for them
- Drunken slumber - A hound in a crib - Getting
awake - The owner of the hound - Sobriety - The
Vienna jug - Another debauch - The exhibition -
The end of the school term - Starting to college at
Cincinnati - My companions - The destruction
wrought by alcohol - Dr. Johnson's declaration
concerning the indulgence of this vice - A warning -
A dangerous fallacy - Byron's inspiration - Lord
Brougham - Sheridan - Sue - Swinburne - Dr.
Carpenter's opinion - An erroneous idea -
Temperance the best aid to thought.

Quit college - Shattered nerves - Summer and
autumn days - Improvement - Picnic parties - A fall
- An untimely storm - Crawford's beer and ale -

Beer brawls - County fairs and their influence on my life - My yoke of white oxen - The "red ribbon" - "One McPhillipps" - How I got home and how I found myself in the morning - My mother's agony - A day of teaching under difficulties - Quiet again - Law studies at Connersville - "Out on a spree" - What a spree means.

Law practice at Rushville - Bright prospects - The blight - From bad to worse - My mother's death - My solemn promise to her - "Broken, oh, God!" - Reflection - My remorse - The memory of my mother - A young man's duty - Blessed are the pure in heart - The grave - Young man, murder not your mother - Rum - A knife which is never red with blood, but which has severed souls and stabbed thousands to death - The desolation and death which are in alcohol.

Blank, black night - Afloat - From place to place - No rest - Struggles - Giving way - One gallon of whisky in twenty-four hours - Plowing corn - Husking corn - My object - All in vain - Old before my time - A wild, oblivious journey - Delirium tremens - The horrors of hell - The pains of the damned - Heavenly hosts - My release - New tortures - Insane wanderings - In the woods - At Mr. Hinchman's - Frozen feet - Drive to town in a buggy surrounded by devils - Fears and sorrows - No rest.

at Indianapolis - At Richmond - The bloated druggist - "Death and damnation" - At the Galt House - The three distinct properties of alcohol - Ten days in Cincinnati - The delirium tremens - My horrible sufferings - The stick that turned to a serpent - A world of devils - Flying in dread - I go to Connersville, Indiana - My condition grows worse - Hell, horrors, and torments - The horrid sights of a drunkard's madness.

Recovery - Trip to Maine - Lecturing in that State - Dr. Reynolds, the "Dare to do right" reformer - Return to Indianapolis - Lecturing - Newspaper extracts - The criticisms of the press - Private letters of encouragement - Friends dear to memory - Sacred names.

At home again - Overwork - Shattered nerves - Downward to hell - Conceive the idea of traveling with some one - Leave Indianapolis on a third tour east in company with Gen. Macauley - Separate from him at Buffalo - I go on to New York alone - Trading clothes for whisky - Delirious wanderings - Jersey City - In the calaboose - Deathly sick - An insane neighbor - Another - In court - "John Dalton" - "Here! your honor" - Discharged - Boston - Drunk - At the residence of Junius Brutus Booth - Lecturing again - Home - Converted - Go to Boston - Attend the Moody and Sankey meetings - Get drunk - Home once more - Committed to the asylum - Reflections - The shadow which whispered "Go away!"

A sleepless night - Try to write on the following day but fail - My friends consult with the officers of the institution - I am discharged - Go to Indianapolis and get drunk - My wanderings and horrible sufferings - Alcohol - The tyrant whom all should slay - What is lost by the drunkard - Is anything gained by the use of liquor? - Never touch it in any form - It leads to ruin and death - Better blow your brains out - My condition at present - The end.

# PREFACE

The days of long prefaces are past. It is also too near the end of the century to indulge in fulsome dedications. I shall, therefore, trouble the reader with only a brief introduction to this imperfect history of an imperfect life. The conditions under which I write necessarily make it lacking in much that would ordinarily have added to its interest. I write within the Indiana Asylum for the Insane; I have not the means of information at hand which I should have to make the work what it should be, and notes which I had taken from time to time, with a view of using them, have unfortunately been lost. Much of my life is a complete blank to me, as I have often, very often, alas! gone for days oblivious to every act and thing, as dead to all about me as the stones of the pavement are dumb. Nor can I connect a succession of incidents one after the other as they occurred in the regular course of my life. The reader is asked to be merciful in his judgment and pardon the imperfections which I fear abound in the book. The title, "FIFTEEN YEARS IN HELL," may, to some, seem irreverent or profane, but let me assure any such that it is the mildest I can find which conveys an idea of the facts. Expect nothing ornate or romantic. The path along which you who walk with me will go is not a flowery one. Its shadows are those of the cypress and yew; its skies are curtained with funereal clouds; its beginning is a gloom and its end is a mad house. But go with me, for you can suffer no harm, and a knowledge of what you will see may lead you to warn others who are in danger of doing as I have done. Unless help comes to me from on high, I feel that I am near the end of my weary and sorrow-laden pilgrimage on earth. You who are in the light, I speak to you from the shadow; you who suffer, I speak to you from the depths; you who are dying, perhaps I may speak to you from the world of the dead; in any case the words herein written are the truth.

Luther Benson

# CHAPTER I

*Early shadows - An unmerciful enemy - The miseries of the curse - Sorrow and gloom - What alcohol robs man of - What it does - What it does not do - Surrounding evils - Blighted homes - A Titan devil - The utterness of the destroyer - A truthful narrative - "It stingeth like an adder."*

Truth, said Lord Byron, is stranger than fiction. He was right, for so it is. Another has declared that if any man should write a faithful history of his own career, the work would be an interesting one. The question now arises, does any man dare to be sufficiently candid to write such a work? Is there no secret baseness he would hide? - no act which, proper to be told, he would swerve from the truth to tell in his own favor? Undoubtedly, many. Doubtless it is well that few have the resolution or inclination to chronicle their faults and failings. How many, too, would shrink from making a public display of their miserable experiences for fear of being accused of glorying in their past shame, or of parading a pride that apes humility. I pretend to no talent, but if a too true story of suffering may interest, and at the same time alarm, I can promise matter enough, and unembellished, too, for no embellishment is needed, as all my sketches are from the life. The incidents will not be found to be consecutive, but set down as certain scenes occur to my recollection - heedless of order, style, or system. Each is a record of shame, suffering, destitution and disgrace. I have all my life stood without and gazed longingly through gateways which relentlessly barred me from the light and warmth and glory, which, though never for me, was shining beyond. From the day that consciousness came to me in this world I have been miserable. In early childhood I swam, as it were, in a dark sea of sorrow whose sad waves forever beat over me with a prophetic wail of desolations and storms to come. During the years of boyhood, when others were thoughtless and full of joy, the sun's rays were hidden from my sight and I groped hopelessly forward, praying in vain for an end of misery. Out of such a boyhood there came - as what else could come? - a manhood all imperfect, clothed with gloom, haunted by horror, and familiar with undefinable terrors which have weighed upon my heart until I have cried to myself that it would break - until I have almost prayed that it would break and thereby free me from the bondage of my pitiless master, Woe! To-day walled within a prison for madmen, looking from a window whose grating is iron, the sole occupant of a room as blank as the leaf of happiness is to me, I abandon every hope. On this side the silence which we call death - that silence which inhabits the dismal grave, there is for me only sorrow and agony keener than has ever before made gray and old before its time the heart of man. Thirty years! and what are they? - what have they been? Patience, and as best I can, I will unfold their record. Thirty years! and I feel that the weight of a world's wretchedness has lain upon me for thrice their number of terrible days! Every effort of my life has been a failure. Surely and steadily the hand of misfortune has crushed me until I have looked forward to my bier as a blessed bed of repose - rest from weariness - forgetfulness of remorse - escape from misery. At the dawn of life, ay, in its very beginning, there came to me a bitter, deadly, unmerciful enemy, accompanied in those days by song and laughter - an enemy that was swift in getting me in his power, and who, when I was once securely his victim, turned all laughter into wailing, and all songs into sobbing, and pressed to my bloated lips his poisonous chalice which I have ever found full of the stinging adders of hell and death. Too well do I know what it is to feel the burning and jagged links of the devil's chain cutting through my quivering flesh to the shrinking bone - to feel my nerves tremble with agony, and my brain burn as if bathed in liquids of fire - too well, I say, do I know what these things are, for I have felt them intensified again and again, ten thousand times. The infinite God alone knows the deep abyss of my sorrow, and help, if help be possible, can come from him alone.

I shall not attempt in these pages any learned disquisition upon the nature of alcohol - its hideous effects on the system - how it disarranges all the functions of the body - how it impairs health - blots out memory, dethrones reason, and destroys the very soul itself - how it gives to the whole body an unnatural and unhealthy action, crucifying the flesh, blood, bones and marrow - how it paints hell in the mind and torture on the heart, and strangles hope with despair.

Nor shall I discuss the terrible and overshadowing evils, financial and social, inflicted by it on every class of society. Like the trail of the serpent it is over all. Look where you will, turn where you may, you can not be blind to its evils. It despoils manhood of all that makes manhood desirable; it plucks hope from the breast of the weeping wife with a hand of ice; it robs the orphan of his bread crumb, and says to the gates of penitentiaries, "Open wide and often to the criminals who became my slaves before they committed crime." The evils of which I speak are not unknown to you, but have you considered them as things real? Have you fought them as present and near dangers? You have heard the wild sounds of drunken revelry mingling with the night winds; you have heard the shrieks and sobs, and seen the streaming, sunken eyes of dying women; you have heard the unprotected and unfriended orphans' cry echoed from a thousand blighted homes and squalid tenements; you have seen the outcast family of the inebriate wandering houseless upon the highways, or shivering on the streets; you have shuddered at the sound of the maniac's scream upon the burdened air; you have beheld the human form divine despoiled of every humanizing attribute, transformed from an angel into a devil; you have seen virtue crushed by vice; the bright eye lose its lustre, the lips their power of articulation; you have seen what was clean become foul, what was upright become crooked, what was high become low - man, first in the order of created things, sunken to a level with brute beasts; and after all these you have or may have said to yourself, "All this is the work of the terrible demon, alcohol."

I shall not attempt to paint any of the countless scenes of degradation, and horror, and misery, which this demon has caused to be enacted. I shall leave without comment the endless train of crimes and vices, the beggary and devastation following the course of this foul Titan devil of ruin and damnation. I shall only endeavor to give a plain, truthful history of one who has felt every pang, every sorrow, every agony, every shame, every remorse, that the demon of drunkenness can inflict. I have nothing to thank this demon for, beyond a few fleeting - oh, how fleeting - hours of false delight. He has wrought only woe and loss to me. Even now, as I sit here in the stillness of desperation, afraid of I know not what, trembling with a strange dread of some impending doom, gazing in fright backward along the shores of the years whereon I see the wrecks of a thousand hopes, the destruction of every noble aspiration, the ruin of every noble resolve, I cry aloud against the utterness of the destroyer. My life has indeed been a sad one; so sad, so lonely, that no language in my power of utterance can give to the reader a full conception of its moonless darkness. Would that the magic pen of a De Quincey were mine that my miseries might stand out until strong-hearted men and true-hearted women would weep, and every young man and maiden also would tremble and turn from everything intoxicating as from the oblivion of eternal death.

To many, certain events which I shall relate in this history may seem incredible; some of the escapes may seem improbable; but again let me assure you that there shall not be one word of exaggeration. The incidents took place just as I shall state them. I have passed through not only all that you will find recorded in these pages, but ten thousand times more. As I lift the dark veil and look back through the black, unlighted past, I shudder and hold my breath as scene after scene, each more appalling than the one just before it, rises like the phantom line of Banquo's issue, defining itself with pitiless distinctness upon my seared eyeballs, until the last and most awful of all stands tall and black by my side, and whispers, hisses, shrieks Madness in my ears. I bow my head and find a moment's relief from the anguish of soul in the hot scalding tears which stream down my fevered cheeks. O God of sure mercy, save other young men from the dark and desolate tortures which gnaw at my heart, and press down upon my weary soul! They are all, all, all the work of alcohol. Oh, how true it is - how true few can understand until their lives are a burden of distress and agony to them - that the cup which inebriates stingeth like an adder. When you see it, turn from it as from a viper. Say to yourself as you turn to fly, "It stingeth like an adder!"

# CHAPTER II

*Birth, parentage, and early education - Early childhood - Early
events - Memory of them vivid - Bitter desolation - An active but
uneasy life - Breaking colts for amusement - Amount of sleep -
Temperament has much to do in the matter of drink - The author
to blame for his misspent life - Inheritances - The excellences of my
father and mother - The road to ruin not wilfully trodden - The
people's indifference to a great danger - My associates - What
became of them - The customs of twenty years ago - What might
have been.*

As to my birth, parentage and education, I am the last but one
of a family of nine children, seven of whom were boys, and all
of whom, excepting one brother, are now living. Both brothers
and sisters are, without an exception, sober, industrious and
honest. I was born in Rush county, Indiana, on the 9th day of
September, 1847.

If there is one spot in all the black waste of desolation about
which I cling with fond memory it is in my early childhood,
and there is no part of my life that is so fresh and vivid as that
embraced in those first early years. I can remember distinctly
events which transpired when I was but two years old, while I
have forgotten thousands of incidents which have occurred
within the past two years. While it is true that in early
childhood a dark shadow fell athwart my pathway, making
everything sombre and painful with an impression of
desolation, yet was my condition happy in comparison with
the rayless and pitchy blackness which subsequently folded its

curtains close about my very being, seeming to make respiration impossible at times and life a nightmare of mockery. Seeming, do I say? Nay, it did, for nothing can be more real than our feelings, no matter how falsely they may be created. The agony of a dream is as keen while it lasts as any other - more so, because there is a helplessness about it which makes it harder to resist.

Many times, lying in my bed after a disgraceful debauch of days' or weeks' duration, has my memory winged its way through the realms of darkness in the mournful and lonesome past, back through years of horror and suffering to the green and holy morning of life, as it at this moment seems to me, and rested for an instant on some quiet hour in that dawn which broke tempestuously, heralding the storms which would later gather and break about me. At such times I could distinctly remember the names and features of all the persons who dwelt in the vicinity of my father's house, although many of them died long ago or passed away from the neighborhood. I could at this time repeat word for word conversations which took place twenty-five years ago. I do not so much attribute this to a retentive memory as to the habit I have had of thinking, when my mind was in a condition to think, of all that was a part of my early life. Again and again, as the years gather up around me, and the valley of life deepens its shadows toward the tomb, do I go back in memory to the days that were. Again and again do I awaken to the beauty, the love, the faces and friends of those days. They are all dear and sacred to me now, though I know they can come no more, and that the hollow spaces of time between the Here and There - the Now and Then - will reverberate forever with the echoes of many-voiced sorrows. Could those who meet me look down into the depths of my ghastly and bitter desolation, they would behold more appalling pictures of human agony than ever mortal eye gazed upon since the opening of the day of time - since the roses of Eden first bloomed and knew not the blight so soon to darken the earthly paradise by the rivers of the east. But I wander from my subject.

I lived and worked on my father's farm until I was eighteen years of age. As I have already said, even when a child I found myself sad and much depressed at times. I could not bear the society of my companions, and at such times would wander away alone to meditate and brood over my misery. At the very threshold of life I was dissatisfied and discontented with my surroundings. I was ever anxious and uneasy, ever longing for some undefinable, unnamable something - I knew not what, but, O God, I knew the desolation of feeling which was then mine. The sorrow of the grave is lighter than that. My life has always been an active one - restless, uneasy, and full of action, I naturally wanted to be doing something or going somewhere. From the time I was seven years old up to the time I was fifteen there was not a calf or colt on the farm that was not thoroughly broken to work or to be ridden. In this work or pastime of breaking in calves and colts I received sundry kicks, wounds, and bruises quite often, and still upon my person are some of the marks imprinted by untamed animals. I only speak of these things that the reader may know the character of my temperament, and thus be enabled to judge more correctly of it when influenced and excited by stimulants which will arouse to rash actions the dullest organizations. I was invariably the last one to go to bed when night came, but not the last to rise, for I always bounded out of bed ahead of the others; and in this connection I can assert with truth that for over twenty years I have not averaged over five hours of sleep out of every twenty-four during that time. I have never found in all nature one object or occupation that gave me more than a swiftly passing gleam of contentment or pleasure. That the reader may clearly comprehend my present condition and impartially judge as to my culpability in certain of my acts, I desire that he may know the circumstances and surroundings of my childhood, for I do solemnly aver that my sorrows and miseries were not of my own planting in those days. While I believe that some men will be drunkards in spite of almost everything that can be done for their relief, others there are, no matter how surrounded, who never will be drunkards, but solely because they abstain from ever tasting the insidious poison. Temperament has much to do with the matter of drink, and could it be known and properly guarded against, I believe that a majority of those having the strongest predisposition to drink, if steps were taken in time, could be saved from its inevitable end, which is madness and death. I would here say to parents that it is their solemn duty to study well the disposition and temperament of their children from the hour of their birth. By proper training and restraint, all wrong impulses might be corrected and the child saved from a life of shameful misery, while they would themselves escape the sorrow which would come to them because of the wrong-doing of the child. While no person is particularly to blame for my misspent life, yet I can clearly see to-day how its worse than wasted years might have been years of use and honor. Its every step might have been planted with actions the memory of which would have been a blessing instead of a remorse.

I have no recollection of a time when I had not an appetite for liquor. My parents and friends of course knew that if it was taken in excess it would lead to destruction, but in our quiet neighborhood, where little was known of its excesses, no one dreamed of the fearful curse which slumbered in it for me to awake. Had they had the least dread, fear, or anticipation of it they would have left nothing undone that being done might have saved me. My appetite for it was born with me, and was as much a part of myself as the air I breathed. There are three kinds of inheritances, some of money and lands, some of superior or great talents, and others of misfortunes. For myself this misfortune was my inheritance. It came not to me directly from my father or mother, but from my mother's father, and seemed to lie waiting for me for three or four generations, and the mistakes and passion of long dead great grandparents reappeared in me, thus fulfilling, with terrible truth, the words of the divine book. It has been gathering strength until when it broke forth its force has become wide-sweeping, irresistible and rushing - a consuming power, devouring and sweeping away whatever dares to arrest its onward progress. Never, never, in those long gone and innocent years of my childhood did my father or mother dream that I, their much-loved child, would ever become a drunkard. If there is anything good, manly, noble or true, that is a part of me, I am indebted to them for it. They loved me, and I worshiped them. The consciousness that I have caused them to suffer so much has been the keenest sorrow of my life. My mother (blessed be the name!) is now in heaven. When she died the light went out from my soul. A pang more poignant than any known before pierced me through and through. My father is living still, and I verily believe there is not a son on earth who more truly and devotedly honors and loves his father than I mine. But I desire to show that I am not wholly responsible for my present unhappy condition. It is natural for every man to wish to excuse, or at least try to soften the lines of his mistakes with palliating reasons, and this I think right so long as the truth is adhered to, and injustice is not done any one. I hope no one will think that I have willfully trod the road to ruin, or sunk myself so low when I have desired the opposite with my whole heart. I was a victim of the fell spirit of alcohol before I realized it. I was raised in a place where opportunities to drink were numerous, as everybody in those days kept liquor, and to drink was not the dangerous and disgraceful thing it's now considered to be. For a radius often miles from our house more people kept whisky in their cupboards or cellars than were without it. I never heard a temperance lecturer until I was twenty years of age, and but seldom heard of one. The people were asleep while a great danger was gathering in the land - a danger which is now known and seen, and which is so vast in its magnitude that the combined strength of all who love peace, order, sobriety and happiness, is scarcely sufficient to meet it in victorious combat.

What associates I had in those days were among men rather than boys, and the men I went with drank. They gave whisky to me and I drank it, and whether they gave it or not, I wanted it. Some of those who gave me drinks are no longer among the living, but neither of them nor of the living would I speak unkindly, nor call up in the memory of one who may read this book a thought that might excite a pang; but I would ask any such just to go back ten, fifteen, and twenty years, and tell me where, are some of the wealthy, influential men of that time?

In the silence of the winding-sheet! How many of them have hastened to death through the agency of whisky? And how few suspected that slowly but surely they were poisoning the wellsprings of life? How many are bankrupts now that might yet be in possession of unincumbered farms, the possessors of peaceful homes, but for that thief accursed - Liquor! Look, too, at some of the sons of these men, and say what you see, for you behold lives wrecked and wretched. Need I tell you what has wrought all this ruin? Need I say that intemperance is at the bottom of it?

The country where I lived in youth and boyhood was equal, if not superior, to any surrounding it. My father's neighbors were all kind-hearted, generous people, and some of them - many of them, indeed - were good Christians, and yet I repeat that twenty years ago there was not a place of a mile in extent but presented the opportunity for drinking. In every little town and village whisky was kept in public and private houses. There was, and yet is, near my father's farm two very small but ancient towns, containing each some twenty or thirty houses, and both of these places have been cursed with saloons in which liquor has been sold for the last thirty years. Both of these towns were favorite resorts with me, especially the one called Raleigh. I have been drunk oftener and longer at a time in Raleigh than in any one place in Indiana. I have written thus of my birthplace and surroundings, that the reader may know the temptations that encompassed me about, and not to speak against any place or people. The country in my father's neighborhood is peopled at this time with noble men and women - prosperous, noted for kindness, generosity, and unpretending virtue. I think if I had been raised where liquor was unknown, and had been taught in early childhood the ruin which follows drinking - if I had had this impressed on my mind, I would have grown up a sober and happy man, notwithstanding my inherited appetite. I would have been a sober man, instead of traversing step by step the downward road of dissipation. I am easily impressed, and in early life might have been taught such lessons as would forever have turned my feet from the wrong and desolation in which they have stumbled so often - in which they have walked so swiftly. Instead of dwelling with shadows of realities the most terrible, and brooding in the cell of a maniac, I might have now communed with the pure and noble of earth.

# CHAPTER III

*The old log school house - My studies and discontent - My first drink of liquor - The companion of my first debauch - One drink always fatal - A horrible slavery - A horseback ride on Sunday - Raleigh - Return home - "Dead drunk" - My parents' shame and sorrow - My own remorse - An unhappy and silent breakfast - The anguish of my mother - Gradual recovery - Resolves and promises - No pleasure in drinking - The system's final craving for liquor - The hopelessness of the drunkard's condition - The resistless power of appetite - Possible escape - The courage required - The three laws - Their violation and man's atonement.*

When I first started to school, log school houses were not yet things of the past, and well do I remember the one which stood near the little stream known as Hood's creek, and Sam Munger, from whom I first received instruction. The next school I attended was in a log house near where Ammon's mill now stands. I attended one or two summer terms at each of these places. There is nothing remarkable connected with my early school-days. They glided onward rapidly enough, but I saw and felt differently, it seemed to me, from those around me; but this may be the experience of others, only I think the melancholy, the fear, the unhappiness which hung over me were not as marked in any one else. I studied but little, because of my discontented and uneasy feeling, but I kept up with my lessons, and have yet one or two prizes bestowed on me twenty years ago for being at the head of my class the greater number of times.

I recollect with painful clearness the first drink of liquor that ever passed my lips. It has been more than twenty-four years since then, but my memory calls it up as if it were only yesterday, with all the circumstances under which I took it. It was in the time of threshing wheat, and then, as in harvesting, log-rolling, and everything that required the cooperation of neighbors, whisky was always more or less used. I was little more than six years of age. A bottle containing liquor was set in the shadow of some sheaves of wheat which stood near a wagon, and taking it I crawled under the wagon with a neighbor now living in Raleigh. We began drinking from this bottle and did not stop until we were both pitiably drunk. The boy who took that first drink with me has since had some experience with the effects of alcohol, but at this time he is bravely fighting the good battle of sobriety and may God always give him the victory. I never could taste liquor without getting drunk. When one drop passed my lips I became wild for another, and another, until my sole thought was how to get enough to satisfy the unquenchable thirst. To-day if I were to dip the point of a needle into whisky and then touch my tongue with that needle, I would be unable to resist the burning desire to drink which that infinitesimal atom would awaken. I would get drunk if hell burst up out of the earth around me - yes, if I could look down into the flames and see men whose eye-brows were burnt off, and whose every hair was a burning, blazing, coiling, hissing snake from their having used the deadly liquid. And if each of these countless fiery snakes had a tongue of forked fire and could be heard to scream for miles, and I knew that another drop would cause them to lick my quivering flesh, yet would I take it. O horror of horrors! I would plunge into the flames forever and ever. After I once taste I am powerless to resist. When I was ten years of age I went one Sunday with a neighbor boy several years older than I, riding on horseback. The course we took was a favorite one with me for it led toward Raleigh, just north of which place I contrived to get a pint or more of the poison called whisky. The doctor from whom I got it had, of course, no idea that I was going to drink it, especially all of it, but drink it I did, getting so completely under its horrible influence that when I arrived at home I fell senseless against the door. My father and mother heard me fall and came out and took me into the house, and just as soon as the heat of the fire began to affect me, I sank into a dead stupor; all consciousness was gone; all feeling was destroyed; all intelligence was obliterated. I lay upon my bed that night wholly oblivious to everything, knowing not, indeed, that such a creature as myself ever existed. The morning came at last, and with it I opened my eyes. Describe who can the thoughts which rushed through my distracted brain. For a little while I knew not where I was or what I had done. My head was throbbing, aching, bursting. I glanced about me and on either side of my bed my father and mother knelt in prayer! Then did I remember what had befallen me, and so keen was my remorse that I thought I would surely die, and, in fact, I wanted to die. O, much loved parents - father on earth and mother in heaven - how often since then have I felt anew the shame of that terrible hour - how often have I seen your sacred faces, wet with the tears of that trial, come before me, looking imploringly heavenward as if beseeching for me the mercy of the infinite God!

That morning the family gathered about the breakfast table, but what a shadow rested over all. A solemnity of silent sorrow was upon us. The peace of yesterday had flown with my return home, and the dark misery of my soul tinged with the shade of the grave's desolation the clouds which were gathering in our sky. O, how often have I prayed that the time might be given back, and that it might be in my power to resist the curse; but the past is implacable as death, and I must bear the tortures that belong to the memory of that most unhappy day. That day, and for many succeeding ones, I read an anguish in the saintly face of my mother that I had never seen there before. My father also bore about with him a look of deep suffering which haunted me for years. For one day I suffered intensely both mentally and physically, but being of a strong, vigorous, and healthy constitution, I was almost completely restored by the following morning. Of course I resolved and promised my father and mother that I would never again taste liquor. For some time I faithfully kept my promise, and for weeks the very thought of liquor was revolting to me. No one becomes a drunkard in a day or week. Alcohol is a subtle poison, and it takes a long time for it to so undermine man's system that he finds life almost intolerable unless stimulated by the hell-broth which must surely destroy him in the end, unless he closes his lips like a vise against it. But for me, I never could drink, from my childhood, without coming under the influence of the accursed poison. I never drank because I liked the taste of liquor, but because I liked the first effects of it. I was never able to tell good liquor or rather pure alcohol - for such a thing as good liquor has never been made - from the worst, the meanest, manufactured from drugs. The latter may be more speedy than pure alcohol, but either will destroy with fatal certainty and rapidity. I drank, as I have said, for the effects, and in the first years of my drinking my first emotions were pleasurable. It sent the blood rushing to the brain, and induced a succession of vivid and pleasing thoughts. But invariably the depression that followed was in the same ratio down as the former was up, and after a time I lost that first pleasant, unnatural feeling, and drank only to satisfy an indescribable passion or craving. At first the wine glass may sparkle and foam, but let it never be forgotten that within that sparkle and foam is concealed the glittering eye of the uncoiled adder. It is the sparkle of a serpent's skin, the foam of the froth of death. Here I must confess that for the past five or six years I have not been able to attain one moment's pleasure from drinking. Every glass that I have touched has proven to be the Dead Sea's fruit of ashes to my lips. I drank wildly, insanely, and became oblivious for days and weeks together to all which was about me, and finally awoke to the horrors which I had sought to drown, but now intensified a thousand fold. No man ever buried sorrow in drunkenness. He can not bury it that way any more than Eugene Aram could bury the body of his victim with the weeds of the morass. Whoever seeks solace in whisky will curse the hour which saw him commit a mistake so fatal. Woe to him who looks for comfort in the intoxicating glass. He will see instead the ghastly face of murdered hope, the distorted vision of a wasted life, his own bloated corpse. The habit of drink after a time becomes more than a mere habit;

Luther Benson

the system comes to demand and crave liquor, it permeates and affects every part of the body until every function refuses to perform its part until it has been aroused to action by its accustomed stimulant.

The most hopeless and wretched slave on earth is he who has bound himself with the fetters of alcohol, and it is a sad and lamentable truth that among thousands very few ever escape from the soul-destroying, health-ruining bondage of an appetite for intoxicating drink. There is only one here and there of all the hosts that are enchained and cursed who succeeds in breaking the bonds which bind body, soul and spirit. So far as the prospect of success is concerned in winning men from evil, I would say, let me go to the brazen-faced and foul-mouthed blasphemer of the holy Master's name; let me go to the forger, who for long years has been using satanic cunning to defraud his fellow-men; let me go to the murderer, who lies in the shadow of the gallows, with red hands dripping with the blood of innocence; but send me not to the lost human shape whose spirit is on fire, and whose flesh is steaming and burning with the flames of hell. And why? Because his will is enthralled in the direst bondage conceivable - his manhood is in the dust, and a demon sits in the chariot of his soul, lashing the fiery steeds of passion to maniacal madness. No possible motive or combination of motives can be urged upon him which will stand a moment before the infernal clamorings of his appetite. Wife, children, home, relatives, reputation, honor, and the hope and prospect of heaven itself, all flee before this fell destroyer. The sufferings and agonies untold of one human soul securely bound by the chains forged by rum are enough to make angels weep and devils laugh. I have no desire to discourage those who have this habit fastened on them. I would not say to them: You can not break away from it. I would do all in my power to aid and strengthen every such person in any attempt he might make to be free. There is escape, but courage is required to make it, and greater courage than has ever been exhibited on the field of battle, amid the thunders of cannon, the roar of deadly conflict, the gleam of sabre and glitter of bayonet. But rather than die the drunkard's death, and go to the drunkard's eternal doom, every drunkard can afford to make this fight. It were better, ten thousand times, that every such one should do as I have done - voluntarily go to an asylum and be restrained until he so far recovers that he can of his own will resist temptation. And there is another aid - a strength stronger than our own - God! He will help every unfortunate one that goes to him in sincerity and humbly implores the divine aid.

I desire here to make a statement in justice to myself. There are three laws, the human, the natural and the divine. You may violate a human law, and the judge, if he sees fit, may pardon your offense. If you violate the divine law, God has prepared a way of escape, and promises pardon on conditions within the reach of all, but for a violation of that which I call natural law, there is no forgiveness. The penalty for every such violation must be, and is, fully paid every time, and while natural laws are as much a part of God's creation as the divine, he would no more set aside a penalty for a violation of one of nature's laws than he would blot out a part of his written word. Yet there are recuperative powers and forces in nature that are wonderful, and there is a spiritual strength that helps us to bear, and overcome, and endure every affliction. I was made a new creature in Christ Jesus at Jeffersonville, Indiana, on the 21st of last January, and had I then gone to work to recuperate and restore by all natural means, my broken body, I am most certain that I never again would have tasted liquor; but instead of using the means God had placed about me, in the supreme ecstacy which comes to a redeemed, a new-born soul, I went to work ten times more laboriously than ever, and soon completely exhausted my bodily strength. My system was drained of every particle of its power to resist the slightest attack of any kind whatsoever, much less to make a successful struggle against my great enemy, and so, physically and mentally exhausted when I was assailed by the black, foul fiend of alcohol, I fell, and fell a second time. I resolved, yea, took an oath the most solemn, that rather than again be overtaken by a disaster so dire, I would have myself entombed within an asylum for the insane. Here at last, I was placed, and here I intend to remain until nature shall restore to my body sufficient strength to resist, with God's help, the next and every attack of my enemy. As God is my witness, I had rather remain within these walls and listen to the cries of the worst maniac here, from day to day, until the last hour of my life - yes, and die and be buried here in the pauper's graveyard, than ever again go out and drink. And now as I close this chapter with a full heart, I go down on my knees in supplication to God for strength and grace to keep me from that which has wrecked all my life and made it a continued round of sorrow and shame. I ask every one who reads this chapter, to pray to God for me with all your heart and soul. Oh! men and women, pray for wretched, miserable, sorrowing, suffering, lonely me.

# CHAPTER IV

*School days at Fairview - My first public outbreak - A schoolmate
— Drive to Falmouth - First drink at Falmouth - Disappointment
- Drive to Smelser's Mills - Hostetter's Bitters - The author's
opinion of patent medicines, bitters especially - Boasting - More
liquor - Difficulty in lighting a cigar - A hound that got in bad
company - Oysters at Falmouth, and what befell us while waiting
for them - Drunken slumber - A hound in a crib - Getting awake
- The owner of the hound - Sobriety - The Vienna jug - Another
debauch - The exhibition - The end of the school term - Starting
to college at Cincinnati - My companions - The destruction
wrought by alcohol - Dr. Johnson's declaration concerning the
indulgence of this vice - A warning - A dangerous fallacy - Byron's
inspiration - Lord Brougham - Sheridan - Sue - Swinburne - Dr.
Carpenter's opinion - An erroneous idea - Temperance the best aid
to thought.*

At the age of sixteen I started to school at Fairview, then as
now, an insignificant but pretty village, some four miles from
where my father lived. William M. Thrasher, at this time
Professor of Mathematics in the Butler University, at
Irvington, near Indianapolis, was the teacher in charge of that
school, and it is to him that I am under obligations for about
all the "book learning" that I possess. True, I went to college
after that, but I merely skimmed over the studies there
assigned me. While at school at Fairview I improved every
opportunity to drink. A fatal instinct guided me to the rum
shop. It was during the first winter of my attendance at the
Fairview school that I was guilty of my first debauch. A young

man from Connersville came over to attend school, and I would remark in passing that his father was chiefly interested in sending him to Fairview because he thought that his boy would here be out of temptation. He arrived at noon one day, and we were immediately made acquainted with each other, an acquaintance which ripened into friendship on the spot. The roads were in good condition for sleighing, and the next morning I proposed a ride. He gladly accepted my invitation, and together we drove to Falmouth. At Falmouth we each took a drink, and this fired us with a desire for more. We drove to a house not far away where liquor was kept by the barrel, and tried to get some, but failed - for we waited and waited to be invited in vain - for no invitation was extended to us. Disappointed and half crazy for whisky, we left the house and started on further in pursuit of the curse. After driving about eight miles we halted at a place called Smelser's Mills, where we were supplied with a bottle of Hostetter's Bitters, which we drank without delay, and which was strong enough to make us reasonably drunk, but which, nevertheless, did not come up to our ideas of what liquor should be. My experience has been that about the worst and cheapest whisky ever sold is that sold under the name of "bitters," and it costs more than the best in the market. Excuse the word "best," but certain parts of Dante's hell are good by comparison. I say to all and every one, shun every drink that intoxicates, and shun nothing quicker than the patent medicines which contain liquor, and while you are about it, shun patent medicines which do not contain liquor. The chances are that they contain a deadlier poison called opium. At any rate they seldom cure and often kill.

After drinking our bottle of poisonous slop - that is, Hostetter's Bitters - my friend and I began to boast, and each labored hard to impress the other with his greatness. In order to make the proper impression, we agreed that it was highly important that we should demonstrate the large quantity we could drink and still be reasonably sober. I knew of a place a few miles further on - a place called Hittle's - where I felt sure I could get whisky without an immediate outlay of cash, a consideration of importance since neither I nor my friend had a penny. We went to Hittle's, and there I was successful in an attempt to get a quart of whisky, which we at once proceeded to mix with the Hostetter article already burning up the lining of our stomachs. The effect was not long in appearing, for in a little while we were both very drunk, and I in particular was in the condition best described as howling, crazy drunk. We stopped at a house to light our cigars - for of course we both smoked and chewed tobacco - and as my friend did not feel like getting out, I reeled into the kitchen and picked up a shovelful of coals, which I lifted so near my mouth that I scorched my hair and burnt my face, and, worse than all, singed the faint suggestion of a mustache that was visible by the aid of a microscope, on my upper lip. While I was engaged in lighting my cigar, a large dog - a tall, lean, much-ribbed, lank and hungry-looking hound - went out to the sleigh, and my friend induced him to accept passage with us; so when I got back to my seat it was proposed that the hound should accompany us. I have often wondered since if he was not heartily ashamed of being seen in our company that day; but we made a martyr of him all the same.

We drove off with a succession of whoops and yells, and carried the hound in front. Our first halt was at Falmouth, where we ordered oysters. The room in which we sat at table was quite small, and a large stove whose sides were red with heat made it uncomfortably hot - especially for us who were already in a sultry state. I had not sat at the table a minute when I fell from my chair against the stove. My leg struck a hinge of the door, and as my friend was too much overcome to realize my condition, I lay there until the hinge burnt a hole through the leg of my pantaloons and then into the flesh. I carry a scar to-day in memory of that time, and the scar is about three inches long. The burn was over half an inch in depth. God only knows what might have been the final result had not assistance soon come in the person of the owner of the house. He called for help, and as soon as it arrived we were placed in our sleigh, and by a kind of instinct drove to Fairview. It was dark by the time we got into Fairview, but we contrived to get our horse within the stable and that unfortunate hound into a corn-crib, in which durance he howled so vigorously that the wild winds which whistled and shrieked around the barn could not be heard for him. His complaining lasted all night, and I do not think any one within a mile of the crib slept that night, my friend and myself excepted. Ay, we slept - slept as I have so often slept since - a slumber as deep and oblivious as death - a drunken sleep, from which we awoke to suffer hell's tortures so justly merited by our conduct. I awoke with a throbbing, aching heart, but by slow degrees did I become conscious that I had been somewhere in a sleigh and done something either very desperate or very foolish, or both. At first my mind was so muddled, so beclouded with the fumes of the infernal "bitters" and whisky that I thought I had burned a city. While I was trying to solve the mystery of my course, I was aided by a revelation so sudden that it startled me, for the owner of the hound came galloping up and fiercely demanded to know where his dog was. He rated us severely - accused us of stealing the animal, and threatened to prosecute us then and there. I knew what we had done. In the meantime some one opened the door of the crib and turned out the hound. He must have recognized the voice of his master, for he joined the latter in his howling, and between them they gave us good reason to wish that our ambition to keep that dog's company had been in vain. The dog was more easily pacified than the man, but finally on our offering to give him three plugs of tobacco to hush up the affair, he became quiet and smoothed the ragged front of his anger. On adding a cigar or two to the plugs, he brightened up and said we might have the "darned houn'" any how, if we wanted him. But we had had enough of his society and were willing to part from him without further expense.

I don't think, seriously speaking, that I ever suffered more keenly from the stings of remorse and fear than I did for one week after this debauch. The remarkable part of it to me was our determination to take the dog. All my life I have disliked dogs - dogs in general and hounds in particular. I resolved never to drink again, and for some time kept the resolution.

A few weeks following this "spree" there was an exhibition at the school house, and several of the larger boys - myself among the number - assembled themselves together, and, after a consultation, decided that, in order to make the exhibition a success, there should be a limited amount of whisky secured for our special use. We took up a collection, each contributing a few cents, and two of the largest, tallest, and stoutest boys were dispatched to Vienna, a small village three miles distant, to get it. A vision of hounds passed before me, but the desire to get a drink drove them yelping out of memory. The boys, on reaching Vienna, bargained for three gallons of liquor, and brought it to our general headquarters. It was wretched stuff - the vilest, meanest, rottenest poison that ever went under the name of whisky. The boys who got it had carried it the three miles by passing a stick through the handle of the jug. They got drunk on the way back with it, and one of them fell into a branch, dragging the jug and the other boy after him. Unfortunately the jug was not broken, and fortunately the boys were not seriously hurt. It was a little after dark when they stumbled across the meeting house yard to where we awaited them. The following day we attacked the contents of the jug, and before midnight we were all drunk - some rather moderately drunk, some very drunk, and some dead drunk, as the phrase is. I myself was of the number that were dead drunk. Some of the boys kept sober enough to fight, but I never would fight, drunk or sober. I do not think I am a coward as regards personal courage, and I really think the fear of hurting others restrained me from ever mixing in brawls in those days.

As the night wore away two or three of the boys became sober enough to hide the jug, which they concealed in a corn-shock. These dragged the rest of us to bed, although one of the party woke up in the wood-box with his head downward and his feet dangling over the top of the box. Only those who have been so unfortunate as to be in a similar condition can realize our state of mental and physical feeling. Parched lips, scalded tongues, cracked throats, throbbing temples, and burning shame were indisputably ours. So we awoke on the morning of the day set apart for the exhibition, an exhibition in which we were to appear before our respected teacher, friends and relatives, besides all the people of the surrounding country. Early in the day we commenced to get ready for the afternoon's work by resorting to the same jug that so recently had bereft us temporarily of reason, and laid us in the mud and snow. I only got one big drink of the poison and so contrived to get through passably well with my part of the performance; some of the boys got too much, and failed to remember anything, so that they failed utterly and hid behind the curtains, and, taken all in all, we did little or nothing toward the success of the exhibition or to making those interested gratified with our parts. Some of the boys who figured on the stage that day are dead; but others are alive and of those I am not the only one writhing in the coils of the serpent of alcohol, though not one of them has fallen so low as I. If at that time I might have been permitted to lift the curtain and looked down future-ward through the unlighted years of shame, and weariness, and suffering, I think the dreadful vision would have stayed me forever in a career which has only grown darker and more unendurable with every step. I kept on much in the same way, increasing in length and frequency my ever recurring debauches, until the end of the school term.

I was well nigh twenty years of age, and from this place went to Cincinnati to attend college. Here the opportunities to gratify my hereditary appetite, made keen and sharp, and ever keener and sharper by indulgence, were all about me. My companions were older and further advanced on the road to ruin than I. My steps were more swift than ever before to tread the path which leads surely to the everlasting bonfire. I could not fail to notice while at college that the most brilliant and intellectual - those whose future prospects were the most pleasing and bright - were the very ones who most frequently drowned their hopes, and sapped their strength and energy in alcoholic stimulants. O, vividly do I recall to mind examples of heaven-bestowed genius, talent, health, and abilities, sacrificed on the worse than bloody teocalli of this hideous and slimy devil, Intemperance! How many master minds, instead of progressing sublimely through the broad, deep, and august channels of thought, became impeded by the meshes and clogs of intoxication, and were thus worse than prevented from exploring the regions of immortal truth! How many dallied with the sirens of the wine cup, until all power to grapple with great subjects was lost irrevocably! How many are the instances in the world's history of great minds debased and ruined by alcohol! Look back and around you at the lives of the brightest literary geniuses and see how many are under the spell of this Circe's baleful power! Think of the rich intelligences whose brightness has prematurely faded and died away in the darkness of alcoholic night! What hopes has alcohol destroyed! What resolves it has broken! What promises it has blighted! Think of any or of all these things, and hasten to say with Dr. Johnson that this vice of drink, if long indulged, will render knowledge useless, wit ridiculous, and genius contemptible. Oh! how many lost sons of earth, whose lamps of genius blazed only to light their pathway to the tomb, might have achieved an inheritance of immortal fame but for this vice, or disease as it may be.

I write this with a hope that it may be a heeded warning to the intellectual of earth, not less than the illiterate. The educated man is more liable to suffer from strong stimulants than the man who is not educated. Never was there a greater or more dangerous fallacy than that so often urged, that the thinking functions are assisted by the use of stimulating liquors or drugs. O, say some, Byron owed a great portion of his inspiration to gin and water, and that was his Hippocrene. Nonsense! His highest inspiration came from the beauty of the world and from God. Lord Brougham, it has been declared, made his most brilliant speeches of old port. Sheridan, it has been told, delivered some of his most sparkling speeches when "half seas over." Eugene Sue found his genius in a bottle of claret; Swinburne in absinthe, and so on. But who shall say what these great, men lost and will lose in the end by this forcing process? Dr. W.B. Carpenter, in referring to the supposed uses of alcohol in sustaining the vital powers, says emphatically that the use of alcoholic stimulants is dangerous and detrimental to the human mind, but admits that its use in most persons is attended with a temporary excitation of mental activity, lighting up the scintillations of genius into a brilliant flame, or assisting in the prolongation of mental effort when the powers of the nervous system would be otherwise exhausted. Concede this, and then answer if it is not on such evidence that the common idea is based that alcohol is a cause of inspiration, or that it supports the system to the endurance of unusual mental labor. The idea is as erroneous as the no less prevalent fallacy that alcoholic stimulants increase the power of physical exertion. Physiologically the fact is established that the depression of the mental energy consequent upon the undue excitement of alcoholic stimulants is no less than the depression of the physical energy following its use. In either case the added strength and exhilaration are of short duration, and the depression and loss exceed the increased energy and the gain. The influence of alcoholic stimulants seems to be chiefly exerted in exciting to activity the creating and combining powers, such as give rise to the high imaginations of the poet and the painter. It is not to be wondered at that men possessing such splendid powers should have recourse to alcoholic stimulants as a means of procuring often temporary exaltation of these powers and of escaping from the seasons of depression to which they and others of less high organizations are subject. Nor is it to be denied that many of these mental productions which are most strongly marked by the inspiration of genius, have been thrown off under the inspiration of the stimulating influences of liquor. But it can not, on the other hand, be doubted that the depression consequent upon the high degree of mental excitement is, as already observed, as great as the first in its way - a depression so great that it sometimes destroys temporarily the power of effort. Hence it does not follow that the authors of the productions in question have really been benefited by the use of these stimulants.

It is the testimony of general experience that where men of genius have habitually had recourse to alcoholic stimulants for the excitement of their powers they have died at an early age, as if in consequence of the premature exhaustion of their nervous energy. Mozart, Burns, Byron, Poe and Chatterton may be cited as remarkable examples of this result. Hence, although their light may have burned with a brighter glow, like a combustible substance in an atmosphere of oxygen, the consumption of material was more rapid, and though it may have shone with a more sober lustre without such aid, we can not but believe that it would have been steadier and less premature without it. We may also doubt that the finest poems and the finest pictures have been written and painted even by those in the habit of drinking while they were under the influence of liquor. We do not usually find that the men most distinguished for a combination of powers called talent or genius, are disposed to make such use of alcoholic stimulants for the purpose of augmenting their mental powers, for that spontaneous activity of mind itself which alcohol has a tendency to excite is not favorable to the exercise of the observing faculties, which are so important to the imagination, nor to those of reason, nor to steady concentration on any given subject, where profound investigation or clear sight is desirable.

Of this we have an illustration in the habit of practical gamblers who, when about to engage in contests requiring the keenest observation and the most sagacious calculation, and involving an important stake, always keep themselves cool either by total abstinence from fermented liquors, or by the use of those of the weakest kind, in very small quantities. We find that the greatest part of that intellectual labor which has most extended the domain of thought and human knowledge has been performed by men of sobriety, many of them having been drinkers of water only. Under this last category may be ranked Demosthenes, Johnson, Haller, Bacon, Milton, Dante, etc. Johnson, it is true, was a great tea drinker. Voltaire drank coffee at times to excess, and occasionally a small quantity of light wine. So, also, did Fontenelle. Newton solaced himself with the fumes of tobacco. Of Locke, whose long life was devoted to constant intellectual labor, who appears independently of his eminence in his special objects of pursuit one of the best informed men of his time, the following explicit testimony is found by one who knew him well: His diet was the same as that of other people, except he usually drank nothing but water, and he thought that his abstinence in this respect had preserved his life so long, although naturally his constitution was so weak. In addition to these examples, which I have quoted at length, I might also mention the case of Cornaro, the old Italian philosopher, who at the age of thirty-five found himself on a bed of misery and imminent death through intemperance. He amended his way of life, and for upwards of four score years after, by a temperate course of living, lived happily and did all the important work which has placed his name among the men of great intellectual powers.

# CHAPTER V

*Quit college - Shattered nerves - Summer and autumn days - Improvement - Picnic parties - A fall - An untimely storm - Crawford's beer and ale - Beer brawls - County fairs and their influence on my life - My yoke of white oxen - The "red ribbon" - "One McPhillipps" - How I got home and how I found myself in the morning - My mother's agony - A day of teaching under difficulties - Quiet again - Law studies at Connersville - "Out on a spree" - What a spree means.*

I left college in the spring of 1866, and returned home to the farm where I spent the summer and autumn months in a very nervous and discontented manner. For over four months my mental condition bordered on that of a maniac, so completely had the use of liquor shattered my nervous system. I became alarmed at my state, and for a time was deterred from drinking, or, if I drank at all, the quantity was small. But fresh air and the little work which I did on the farm, soon restored me. As the summer wore away I attended pleasure parties, and found, not happiness, but a moment's forgetfulness among the merry picnic parties in the woods. I had also the distinguished honor of actually superintending and presiding over two of these festivities, both of which were held in Horace Elwell's woods, on the unsung, but classically rustic banks of Tom. Hall's mill-dam, near the village which bears the historic and great name of Raleigh. I succeeded in tiding myself through the first picnic without getting drunk. I mean more particularly that I remained sober during the day - that is, sober enough to keep it from being known that I had drank more than once or twice; but that night at the ball at Louisville, I bit the dust, or, to get at the truth more literally and unrhetorically, I fell down stairs and came within a point of breaking my neck. Had I been sober the fall would have put an end then and there to my miserable and worthless existence; but lest any one should argue from this that after all whisky sometimes saves life, I would have them bear in mind that if I had been sober the chances are I would not have fallen.

The next picnic was sadly interfered with by a violent storm of wind and rain, which came up the day before the one set apart for it. The water washed the sawdust which had been sprinkled on the ground for the dancers' benefit into Hall's fretful mill-race, and thence down into the turbulent and swollen Flat Rock. This, as well as other creeks, became so high that it was out of the question to ford them. The boys could get to the grounds very well, and many of them did get there, but the girls were not of a mind to risk their lives for a day's doubtful amusement, and so the picnic failed in the beginning. The young men - myself, of course, in the lot - determined to have what was called "fun" at any rate, and to this end they congregated during the day at Raleigh. Mr. Sam Crawford had an abundant supply of beer and ale, and I wish to say that if there are any persons so innocent as to doubt that beer and ale intoxicate they would change from doubt to faith in the power of these slops to make men drunk, could they experience or see what took place at Raleigh on that day. They would be willing to testify in any court that beer will not only intoxicate, but, taken in sufficient quantities, it will make men beastly drunk and fill them with a spirit of fiendish cruelty. There were on that day as many as four fights, with enough miscellaneous howling, cursing and billingsgate to fill out the natural make-up of a hundred more. I was drunk - so drunk that I did not know at the last whether my name was Benson or Bennington. I suppose I would have sworn to the latter, had the question been raised, but it was not. I did not fight, for, as I have said, I seemed to have an instinctive dread of doing something terrible in the event of my getting engaged in combat with another. Like Falstaff, it may be, I was a coward on instinct. I have always thought, moreover, that the Hudibrastic aphorism is worthy of practice, because nothing can be more evident than the fact that

" - He who runs away
May live to fight another day."

From that time to the commencement of the season for county fairs, five or six weeks later, I kept in a condition of sobriety. County fairs, I wish to say, and especially the Rush county fairs, did more toward bringing on the disastrous career which has been mine - a career which has befouled the record of my life and marked almost every page of its history - witness this biography - with blots of shame, discord and unholy suffering than any other cause of an external character. I was very young when I first commenced to take stock to the fair to exhibit for premiums. I always went on the first day, and always remained until the fair came to a close, staying on the grounds night and day. There was a vagabond element in my nature which harmonized perfectly with this sort of life. The men with whom I associated were, in general, of that class who like liquor alone or in company, and each had his jug of favorite whisky, which was supposed to be a sure preventive against cold and colds in cold weather, and against heat and fever in hot weather. If invited to drink the rule was to accept immediately and return the courtesy as soon as convenient.

In those days I was the proud possessor of a yoke of white oxen, and I made it a point to exhibit them at every fair within my reach, for they invariably won the Red Ribbon, then a mark of the first prize. Alas, that it did not mean to me what it now does! It meant anything rather than total abstinence; it was an unfailing sign of drunkenness; it told of shameful revels, of days of debauchery and nights of misery when not passed in beastly slumber. That ribbon is now a symbol of holy temperance - it was then a souvenir of days of disorder and evil-doing.

During the winter I was engaged to teach a district school, and for three months managed to keep tolerably sober - that is, I did not get drunk more than three or four times, and then on Saturday nights and Sundays. One Sunday - it was the coldest day that winter - I went to Falmouth and visited a drinking place kept by one McPhillipps. While there I drank eleven glasses of whisky. At nine o'clock in the evening, I can indistinctly remember, I mounted my horse and started home, and from that moment until the next day I knew nothing whatever that took place. From the way I was bruised and battered I judge that I must have struck almost every fence corner between McPhillipps' place and home. My legs were in a woful plight, and having turned black and blue, they were frightful to see. On arriving at the gate which led into the front yard at home, I fell off my horse and tumbled to the ground, a wretched heap of helpless clay. I remained on the ground, lying in the snow, until I froze my hands, feet, and ears. It was about three o'clock in the morning when I got to the house. So they told me, for I have no knowledge of going, and, indeed, I remembered nothing that took place.

When I came to consciousness I found myself wrapped up in a blanket, lying in bed, with hot bricks at my feet. I was in the room occupied by father and mother, and the first object that met my wandering sight was the face of my mother. The look with which she regarded me will never fade from my memory. There was in it the sorrow and anguish of death. She rose from her bed at sight of me, and with streaming eyes and screaming voice called the family up to bid them good-by; she said she was dying - that I had killed her. I sprang from my bed in such a horror of terrible suffering, mental and physical, as never swept over the body and soul of mortal man. I felt my heart thumping and beating as though it would burst forth from my bosom; the hot, hissing blood rushed to my aching, fevered brain, and a torrent of sweat burst forth on my icy forehead. I could not have suffered more physical agony had a thousand swords been driven through my quivering body, nor would my miserable soul have been in more insufferable pain had it been confined in the regions of the damned. It was some time before anything like quiet was restored, but as soon as it was, some of the family went to the gate and found my hat and took charge of the horse which I had ridden. That morning I dragged myself to school with a sad, heavy heart. As my scholars came in, they seemed to understand that something was the matter with me, and often during the day their wondering looks were directed toward me as if they sought some explanation of my appearance. The day was a long and weary one to me - a day, like many another since then, of most intense wretchedness. About noon one of my feet became so swollen that it was necessary for me to take off my boot, and by the time I dismissed school it had got so bad that I could not draw on my boot, so that I had to walk home, a distance of one mile, over the frozen ground with nothing to protect my foot but a woolen sock. On entering the house, my mother burst into tears at sight of me. I must have been a pitiable object, and yet how little did I deserve the wealth of priceless sympathy lavished upon me. That night, and many nights succeeding it, the only way I could get into bed was to put an old-fashioned chair with rounds in the back, beside the bed and crawl up round by round until I got on a level with the bed, and then let go and fall over into the bed.

It is needless for me to say that I firmly resolved and honestly felt that I would never again taste the liquor which leads to madness, misery, and death. For some time I kept my resolution; and would to God that I could here conclude by saying that I never again allowed a drop of it to pass my lips. But I am writing an autobiography, and I have told you that I would not shrink from telling the truth. So it will happen that other and still more desperate and disgraceful episodes of drunkenness will have to be recorded.

In the spring of 1867 I went to Connersville, and began the study of law with the Hon. John S. Reid. Unfortunately, and I fear designedly, I made my acquaintances among, and selected my companions from, the most dissolute, idle, and intemperate class of young men in the town. Connersville then had and still has among its citizens some very wealthy men, who suffered their boys to grow up without much care, mostly in idleness. As might be expected the indifference of the fathers, joined to the natural inclinations of the sons, has proved the ruin of the latter. I now call to mind several of those young men who are hopeless and complete wrecks. Idleness and dissipation have done their terrible work in every case which I call to mind.

I read a little law, and drank a great deal of whisky, and as a natural consequence the time then passing was for the most part worse than lost. Up to this period the duration of my sprees was not longer than a day and night. They now were not confined to one day, for when I went out on what is called a "regular spree," it was liable to be two or three days, as it has since been two or three weeks, before I got back. Got back! Where from? The reader knows too well.

Out on a spree! These are melancholy and heart-breaking words. Out on a spree! Oh, how much of misery is implied! Out on a spree! Readers, every one, I hope you will never have it said that you are out on a spree. To go out on a spree is to throw away strength, without which the battle of life can not be fought; it is to squander money which you may need badly for the necessaries of life, which had better be thrown into the fire and burnt up than spent in such a way; it is to quench the light of ambition, to crush hope, entomb joy, lay waste the powers of the mind, neglect duty, desert the family, and commit in the end suicide. Arson may have walked by your side while out on a spree, red murder may have grinned, dagger in hand, upon you, and death stalked within your shadow, ready in a thousand ways to strike you down. Don't go out on sprees. Think of the pity of them, the wrong, the disgrace, the remorse, the misery. Going on an occasional spree only will not do. Some men will keep sober for weeks, and even months, but a birthday, or a wedding, or a national holiday, or a fit of the blues, or a streak of good luck, starts them off, and habit, like a smouldering flame, breaks out, and for a time all is over. Such men scotch, but they do not kill the cobra of intemperance, and soon or late the other result will follow, the snake will kill them. The reptile is tenacious of life, and so long as the life remains there is danger from the deadly venom of its tooth. Those who have never formed the habit of drinking had better die at once than live to form it. Those who have formed the habit should subdue it and never enter into a compromise with it. The good effects of months of abstinence may be swept away in an hour. Open the flood-gates of indulgence never so little and the torrent will force its way through and drown every worthy resolution. Its tide is next to resistless. Days of drunkenness succeed, months of self-denial are lost, and deplorable results follow everywhere. Wives are driven to desperation, mothers to despair, children to want. Demoralization, starvation, damnation follow. Friends are separated, homes are desolated, and souls are driven to hell itself, and yet people will talk lightly, and even jokingly of the very thing which leads to these terrible losses and sufferings - out on a spree.

Debauches not only destroy all capacity for usefulness while they last, but they demand the vital strength which has wisely been gathered in the system for days of possible need, when sickness and natural infirmities will lay hands on the mind or body. The debauch of to-day will borrow from to-morrow or from next week, or month, or year, that which can not be restored. The bloated face, the dull, glassy eye, the furtive glance of fear and shame, the trembling gait, all speak of ravages produced by other causes than those of time. Indeed, the flight of years can produce no such effects, for inexorable and wearing as fleeting days and months are, their natural results differ very widely from those which are caused by an abuse of the powers of nature. Besides this, many men who are shattered wrecks are still young in years, and the dew of youth but for dissipation might yet have glistened on their foreheads.

It was at this period that the appetite burst forth in a fearful flame which scorched life itself, and burnt every energy of my being. It was fast getting to be a consuming, craving, devouring passion, subjecting my very soul to its dreadful tyranny. My spells increased in frequency, and their duration was more and more prolonged. I would remain drunk from eight to ten days, until I got so nervous that I could not sleep, and night after night I would be counting the hours and longing for morning, which, when it came with its blessed light, gradually revealing the pattern of the paper on the walls, caused me to hide my face in the bedclothes and wish for black and never-ending night to come and hide me from the world and my misery. From such vigils, feverish and unrefreshed, it may easily be supposed that I sought the open window in anguish, and bathed my aching, throbbing forehead in the cool, pure air. At last my condition became so deplorable that my friends sent my father word to come and take me home, which he did. While at Connersville, in all my dark and desolate trials, William Beck was my friend and helper. He never then forsook me, and he never since has forsaken me, but still remains my faithful and sympathizing friend - a friend whose valuation is beyond gold, and for whom I entertain the deepest feelings of gratitude. I returned home with my father and remained several months, keeping sober all the while. During most of the time I applied myself vigorously to the study of the law, making rapid progress.

I believe I have as yet not stated that, in the intervals long or short between my sprees, I abstained totally from the use of ardent spirits. I never could and never did drink in moderation. One drink would always kindle such a fire in my blood that it was out of my power to prevent its spreading into a conflagration. I have very many times been accused of "drinking on the sly," as they say, but every such accusation is false. I have also been accused of using opium. I know the pitiable wretch that started that lie - for it is a lie - and the poor dupe that repeated it. For five years my appetite has been so fierce at times, that, I repeat, had I touched the point of the finest needle in alcohol and placed it to my tongue, I would have got drunk had I known that that drunk would have plunged my soul into hell and eternal torments. O appetite, cold, cruel, heartless, accursed, consuming, devouring appetite! No other malady like thee ever afflicted man. Would that I could paint thee, in all thy accursed hideousness, in letters of unfading fire, and write them in the vaulted firmament to flame forth to all generations to come their eternal warning.

Luther Benson

# CHAPTER VI

*Law Practice at Rushville - Bright prospects - The blight - From bad to worse - My mother's death - My solemn promise to her - "Broken, oh, God!" - Reflection - My remorse - The memory of my mother - A young man's duty - Blessed are the pure in heart - The grave - Young man, murder not your mother - Rum - A knife which is never red with blood, but which has severed souls and stabbed thousands to death - The desolation and death which are in alcohol.*

My next move was to Rushville, where I opened an office and commenced practicing law. For a time I kept sober, and was so successful in my profession that from the very beginning I more than made my expenses. In fact my prospects for a brilliant career as a lawyer seemed most flattering. The predictions were many that an uncommon future lay before me, but, alas, I could stand prosperity no better than adversity. My appetite grew to such a craving for stimulants that it tortured me. It had slumbered for weeks, as it has since, only to make itself manifest in the end with the force of a hurricane. While it had appeared to sleep it was gathering strength. At the time it dragged me down I was boarding with some others at the house of an elderly widow. So completely was I transformed from a man into something debased that I went to her house and fell through the front door on the floor dead drunk. The landlady had me carried back to my office, where I lay like a water-sodden log, wholly unconscious, until the next morning. When I awoke I had no knowledge of anything that had happened. My friends informed me of my fall at the house, and of their bearing me back to the office. I upbraided myself bitterly, but it was days before I had the courage to show my face on the streets, so keen were my shame and sense of disgrace. Time softens the wildest remorse, and in a few weeks I regained a state of quiet feeling. But unfortunately most of my associates were among the class of young men who are never averse to taking a drink, and it was not long before I found myself again visiting the saloons, although I did not give up right away to take a drink with them. But I got to staying in the saloons more than in my office, and began to go down steadily. Good people who felt sorry for me, and who wanted to aid me, would do nothing for me unless I would do something for myself, and this I could not, or did not do.

I moved from office to office, always descending in respectability, because always violating my promises not to drink. Occasionally I would make a desperate effort to reform, gathering about me every element of strength which I could possibly command, and for a while I would be successful, but just as hope would begin to light up my darkened path and my friends begin to feel a new-born confidence in me, an infernal and terrible desire would take possession of me, and in a moment all that I had gained would be swept away by my yielding to the demon that tempted me. A debauch longer and more utterly sickening and vile than the last followed, after which I would settle down into a condition of hopelessness which would appal the bravest and strongest. So deplorable, indeed, was my feeling regarding the matter that then, as since, I kept on drinking for days after the appetite had left me or had been satiated, in order to deaden the horrible agony that I knew would crush me when my reason returned.

I now come to an event in my life which affected me at the time beyond the power of words, and which I can not without tears of choking sorrow even now dwell upon. I refer to the death of my mother, which occurred during the winter after my going to Rushville in 1867. She had been sick a long time, and had suffered very intense pain, but for days before her death I think she forgot her own physical torments in anxiety and solicitude about me. I went home a few days before she died, and remained with her until the last. She talked to me much and often, always begging and pleading with me as only a dying mother can plead, to save myself from the life of a drunkard. I promised her solemnly and honestly that I would never again taste liquor. As I gazed upon her wasted face and read death in every lineament, and heard the dread angel's approach in every breath of pain she drew, and saw above all in her fast dimming eye that the horrors of her approaching dissolution were almost unthought of in her care for me, I resolved deep down in my heart never to taste liquor again, and kneeling by her dying form, I called heaven to witness that no more, oh, never, never more, would I go in the way of the drunkard, or touch, in any form, the unpitying and soul-destroying curse. I looked on her face, which was growing strangely calm and white. She was dead, and it came upon me that she who had loved and suffered most for me, and without a reproach, was never more to look upon me again or speak words of comfort and aid to my ears, so often unheeding. At that moment, looking through scalding tears at her holy face, and afterwards when I heard the grave clods falling with their terrible sound upon her coffin lid, I swore that I would keep my promise, no matter what the temptation to break it might be. She would not be here to see my triumph, but I would conquer for her memory's sake, and all would be well. I swore by earth, sea, and sky, never, never to break the promise made to her in the moment of her dying. That promise I broke within two months from the day it was solemnized by my mother's death. I shudder still, remembering the agony of that fall. Broken, oh God! - the promise has been broken, is what first entered my mind. Never before had I suffered as I then suffered.

My wild revel was protracted for days out of dread of the awful sorrow and remorse that I knew must surely come on my getting sober. My mother appeared to me in my troubled dreams, and talked to me as in life. Many times in my slumber, and in my waking fancies did I see her pale, troubled face, with her pitying eyes looking on me as from that bed of pain and death, and at such times I reached out my hands toward her in mute pleading for forgiveness, forgetting or not knowing that she was dead. But the moment soon came when the truth was flashed through the blackness of night upon me, and then my misery was more than I could bear. For years before her death I had lain in my bed and listened to her moaning in her troubled sleep, to the sighs which escaped from her heart and that of my father, and I promised the God of my hoped-for salvation that if he would only let me live I would no more give them pain. Cold, clammy sweat broke out over my face, and my heart beat so low, and slow, and weak, that in very terror I felt that my eyeballs were bursting from my head. Again and again I begged, and plead, and prayed that God would spare me and let me live until I could convince my father and mother that I never would drink again. But my prayers were not answered. My mother went out from me in fear, and dread, and doubt. My father lives, but for me he has little or no hope. If ever a mortal longed and yearned for one thing more than another in this uncertain existence, I long for a peaceful and quiet evening of life for my beloved father. I implore the Father of all of us to give me grace and strength enough to keep sober until my remaining parent is fully persuaded that I am truly and beyond question saved from the curse which has driven me to an asylum, and well nigh sent him, a broken-hearted man, to his grave. O for a strength which will forever enable me to resist the hell-born and hell-supported power of the fiend Alcohol! Could I do this and have my father know it his dying hour would be full of sweet peace, and a joy so shining that its light would drive afar off the shadows of his death agony. In that knowledge death would be vanquished and heaven would stoop to earth and cover his grave with glory. Oh, God! Grant me this one boon! Give me this one request! In every step of my life I have disappointed him. In the future let all other hopes, and joys, and aspirations die, if needs be, all but this - this one - that I may never in any way touch liquor again. May every man and woman who sees this allow their hearts to go out in an earnest prayer that I may succeed in this one thing. It is now too late for me to reach the bright promises of other years. It is now too late for me to regain all that has been lost, but this I would do, and it will make me feel at the last that I have not lived altogether to be a remorse and shame to those who are bound to me by ties which can not be broken. God may answer your prayers if not mine, so that from the throne of heavenly grace may come the peace and rest for which my weary soul has sought so long in vain.

When I drank after my mother's death, many persons took occasion, on learning of it, to censure me in unsparing terms. It was even said that I did not love my mother in life, that I had no respect for her memory in death, and that I was a heartless wretch. These persons had no knowledge of the power of my appetite. They did not know that the passion for liquor, once developed or firmly established, is stronger in its unholy energy than the love of the heart - of my heart, at least - for mother, father, brother, or sister. But let me beg that I may not be charged with indifference to my mother's memory. She comes before me now; she who was a true wife, a faithful friend, a loving and gentle mother, and I kneel to her and pray her blessing and pardon - I would clasp her to my heart, but alas! when I would touch her, the bitter memory comes that she is gone. But I would not repine, for I know she is with her God. Her life was pure and blameless, and her soul, on leaving its weary earthly tabernacle, passed to its inheritance - a mansion incorruptible, and one that will not fade away. She bore her cross without a murmer of complaint, and she has been crowned where the spirit of the just are made perfect. Blessed are the pure in heart, we read, and I know that I am not misquoting the spirit of the holy book when I say for the same reason, blessed is my mother, for she was pure of heart, and passed from tribulation to peace, from night to day, from sorrow to joy, from weariness to rest - rest in the bosom of God.

It may be that some young man will read these pages whose mother is still among the living. I do not think that such a one will be without love for his mother - a dear, compassionate, doating, gentle mother, who loved him before he knew the name of love; who sang him to sleep in the years that were, and awoke him with kisses on the bright mornings long ago; who bathed his head with a soft hand when it throbbed with pain, and smiled when the glow of health was on his cheek. She wept holy tears when he suffered, and when he was delighted her heart beat with pleasure. It was she who taught him that august prayer which is sacred in its simplicity to childhood. She is aged now; her wealth of brown hair is white with age's winter, her step is no longer quick, her eye has lost its lustre, and her hand is shaken with the palsy of lost vigor. There are wrinkles in her brow and hollows in the cheeks which were once so lovely that his father would have bartered a kingdom for them. She is sitting by the side of the tomb waiting for the mysterious summons which must soon come. Oh, young man, you for whom this mother has suffered, you for whom she cherishes a love which is priceless and deathless, you will not hasten her into eternity by an act, or word, or look, will you? It would kill her to know that you had fallen under sin's destroying stroke. Sometimes she goes to the portrait of your boyish face and looks at it; at other times she takes down some worn and faded garment, that you were wont to wear in those beautiful days of the past, and recalls how you looked when you wore it; then she goes to the room where you used to sleep and looks at the cradle in which she so often rocked you to sleep, and, after all is seen, she returns to her chair - the old easy chair - and waits to hear tidings of you. What would you have her know?

What news of yourself can you send her? Think of it well. Will you put your wayward foot on her tender and feeble heart? Is her breathing so easy that you would impede it with a brutal stab? Oh, if you know no pity for yourself, have some for her. You will not murder her, will you? Yes, you reply, and the laughter of mocking devils floats up from the caves of hell - "Yes! give me more rum!" Now, hear the truth: The time will come when the grass will seem to wither from your feet, pain will stifle your breath, remorse will gnaw your heart and fill all your days and nights with misery unspeakable; your dreams will torture you in sleep, and your waking thoughts will be torments; your path will lie in gloom, and your bed will be a pillow of thorns. You will cry in vain for that departed mother. You will beg heaven to give her back, but the grave will be silent. The grasses are creeping over her tomb, and the white hands have crumbled upon her faithful breast. But no, you will not kill her. You will not call for rum. I have wronged you, thank God! You will be a man. You are a man. You will lay this book down, and swear that you will never touch the accursed, ruinous drink, and you will keep your oath. By sobriety and good habits you will lengthen your mother's days in the land, and smooth her troubled brow, and give strength to her failing limbs.

Rum is a dreadful knife whose edge is never red with blood, but which yet severs throats from ear to ear. It assassinates the peace of families, it cuts away honor from the family name, it lets out the vital spark of life, and is followed by inconsolable death. It pierces hearts, and enters the bosom of trust, goring it with gashes which God alone can heal. Rum is a robber who is deaf to hungry children's cries and famished wives' pleadings. He is a fell destroyer from whom peace and comfort and content fly. No one can afford to be his subject, and it is the duty of every one to rise in arms against him. Let him be cursed everywhere. Let anathemas be hurled against him by the young and old of both sexes. Death is an angel of mercy sometimes - this destroyer never. Death may open the gates of heaven to every victim, but this destroyer can unbar alone the gates of hell. He takes away concord and love and joy, and in their stead leaves the horror and misery of pandemonium!

# CHAPTER VII

*Blank, black night - Afloat - From place to place - No rest - Struggles - Giving way - One gallon of whisky in twenty-four hours - Plowing corn - Husking corn - My object - All in vain - Old before my time - A wild, oblivious journey - Delirium tremens - The horrors of hell - The pains of the damned - Heavenly hosts - My release - New tortures - Insane wanderings - In the woods - At Mr. Hinchman's - Frozen feet - Drive to town in a buggy surrounded by devils - Fears and sorrows - No rest.*

From this time until I tried to break the terrible chain that bound me by lecturing on the miseries and evils of intemperance, my life was one long, hopeless, blank, black night. More than one half of the time for five years I was dead to everything but my own despairing, helpless, pitiable and despicable condition. I was afloat without provision, sail, or compass, on an ocean of darkness, and from one period of deeper gloom to another I expected to go down in the sightless oblivion and so end my accursed existence. I could see no prospect of a rift in the curtain of pitchy cloud which hung over me. I was myself an ever-shifting, restless, uneasy tempest. My unrest and nervous dread of some swift approaching doom too awful to be conceived became so intense and real that I fled from place to place. Not unfrequently I came to myself during these epochs of madness and found that I was a hundred or more miles from home, without friends, respectable or even sufficient clothing, or money - a bloated and beastly wreck. I know not how I ever found my way back, or why I prolonged my life under such circumstances; but it seems the instinct called self-preservation was yet stronger than the ills which assailed me. Days were like weeks to me, and weeks as months, and mouths as years, and in all and through all I managed to crawl forward toward the grave which is still out yonder in the future, finding no pleasure in myself and no delight in anything beautiful and holy. As I lift the dread curtain and glance tremblingly along the path which stretches through the funereal shadows of the past, I feel that it was a thousand years ago when I was a child in my mother's dear protecting arms. Sin may have moments of pleasure, but the pleasure is but a hollow semblance in advance of seemingly never-ending hours of remorse and suffering.

More than once I made desperate efforts to escape from my humiliating thraldom, and, as I was sober during the days of struggle, I sought and found business, and thus managed to secure a little money, although most of my clients were poor and anything but influential. I always did my best for them, however, and seldom lost a case. But at the end of a few days a strange, undefinable, uneasy feeling began to crawl over me and crept into my heart; I became more and more restless, anxious and nervous. I was soon too uneasy to sit still or lie down. Horrible sufferings, agonies untold, woe unspeakable, deprived me of reason, and when I had the inclination I had not the will to guide myself aright. Then all of a sudden, my fierce and unrelenting appetite would sweep, vulture like, down upon me, and I would feel myself on the point of giving way. After this I would rally for a brief season, but only to sink into still deeper misery and desperation. There were days without food, and nights without sleep, but - God pity me! - not without liquor. I lived on the hellish liquid alone, and such a life! The devils of the lower world could see nothing to envy in it. It was worse than their own torture. The quantity of liquor which I now required was enormous. I have drank, on the closing days of a spree, one gallon of whisky within the duration of twenty-four hours, and when I could not get whisky, I would drink alcohol, vinegar, camphor, liniment, pepper-sauce - in short, anything that would have a tendency to heat my stomach. I would have drank fire could I have done so knowing that it would satisfy the thirst that was consuming me. I left untried no means that would enable me to break away from my appetite. For two or three summers after I began practicing law, I went into the country and engaged myself to plow corn at seventy-five cents per day, in order to keep myself as long as possible from the dangers of the town. In the autumn season, after a debauch of weeks, I have hired out and shucked or husked corn in order to get money with which to buy myself boots and winter clothing. I occasionally taught school in the country, but not for money, for I have made more at my profession, when in a condition to practice it, in a single day than I got for teaching a whole month. My object was to free myself, to break my manacles, to open the door of my prison cell and walk forth in the upright posture of a man. Sadly I write, "in vain!" If I fled, the demon outran me; if I broke a link, the demon moulded another; if I prayed, he put the curse into my mouth. As I look back over my horror-haunted, broken, misspent, and false existence, I realize how worthless I am, and I see that my life is a failure. I am in my thirty-second year, and am prematurely old, without the wisdom, or gray hairs, or goodness, or truth, or respect which should accompany age. My heart is frosty but not my hair.

I will now endeavor to recite some of the scenes through which I passed, that the reader may form for himself an opinion regarding my sufferings. I left Rushville on one of my periodical sprees (I do not remember the exact time, but no matter about that, the fact is burning in my memory), and after three or four weeks of blind, insane, drunken, unpremeditated travel - heaven only knows where - I found myself again in Rushville, but more dead than alive. I experienced a not unfamiliar but most strange foreboding that some terrible calamity was impending. I was more nervous than ever before, so much so in fact that I became alarmed seriously, and called on Dr. Moffitt for medical advice. He diagnosed my case, and informed me that my condition was dangerous, unnatural and wild. He gave me some medicine and kindly advised me to go into his house and lie down, I remained there two days and nights, and in spite of his able treatment and constant care I grew worse. Do you know what is meant by delirium tremens, reader? If not, I pray God you may never know more than you may learn from these pages. I pray God that you may never experience in any form any of the disease's horrors. It was this, the most terrible malady that ever tortured man, that was laying its ghastly, livid, serpentine hands upon me. All at once, and without further warning, my reason forsook me altogether, and I started from Dr. Moffitt's house to go to my boarding place. The sidewalks were to me one mass of living, moving, howling, and ferocious animals. Bears, lions, tigers, wolves, jaguars, leopards, pumas - all wild beasts of all climes - were frothing at the mouth around me and striving to get to me. Recollect that while all this was hallucination, it was just as real as if it had been an undeniable and awful reality. Above and all around me I heard screams and threatening voices. At every step I fell over or against some furious animal. When I finally reached the door leading to my room and just as I was about to enter, a human corpse sprang into the doorway. It had motion, but I knew that it was a tenant of that dark and windowless abode, the grave. It opened full upon me its dull, glassy, lustreless eyes; stark, cold, and hideous it stood before me. It lifted a stiffened arm and struck me a blow in the face with its icy and almost fleshless hand from which reptiles fell and writhed at my feet. I turned to rush into another room, but the door was bolted. I then thought for a second that I was dreaming, and I awoke and laughed a wild laugh, which ended in a shriek, for I knew that I was awake. I turned again toward my own door, and the form had vanished. I jumped into my room and tore off my clothes, but as I threw aside my garments, each separate piece turned into something miscreated and horrible, with fiendish and burning eyes, that caused my own to start from their sockets. My room was filled with menacing voices, and just then a mighty wind rushed past my window, and out of the wind came cries, and lamentations, and curses, which took shapes unearthly, and ranged about the bed on which I lay shuddering. Die! die! die! They shrieked. I was commanded to hold my breath, and they threatened horrors unimaginable if I did not obey.

I now believed that my time had come to render up the life which had been so much abused. I asked what would become of my soul when my body gave it up, and they told me it would descend to the tortures of an everlasting hell, and that once there, my present sufferings would be as bliss compared with what was in store for me for an endless age. As my eyes wandered about the room - I was afraid to close them - I saw that innumerable devils were crowding into it. They were henceforth to be my companions, and if the Prince of all of them ever allowed me to leave for a brief time the regions of infernal woe, it would be in their company and on missions such as they were now fulfilling. I called aloud for my mother, and a voice more diabolical than any I had yet heard, hissed into my ears that she was chained in hell, but immediately a million devils screamed, "Liar! she is in heaven!" I refused then to hold my breath, and told them to kill me and do their worst. In an instant the spirit of my mother, like a benediction, rested beside me. As she begged for me I knew that it was her voice, natural as in her life on earth. While she was yet imploring for me the room became radiant, and I saw that it was full of angels. I felt a strange joy. My sins were pardoned, and I was told that I should go forth and preach and save souls. I was commanded to get out of bed, put on my clothes, and go down stairs, where I would be told what to do. I obeyed, and on opening the door that led to the street, a man came to me and he bid me follow him. The spirits whispered to me that the man was Christ, and his looks, acts and steps even were such as I had conceived were his when he was once a meek and lowly sufferer on earth. I followed him about sixty rods, when he told me to stop. I did so, and just then the heavens opened with a great blaze of glory, and millions of angels came down. Such music as then broke upon my senses I never heard before, and have never since heard. The angels would approach near me and tell me they were going to take me to heaven with them; then they would disappear for an instant and devils gathered about me. I could hear music and see the heavenly hosts returning. They came and went many times thus, and after they went away the last time, I was again surrounded by fiends who inflicted every torture on me. Christ commanded me to stand in that place, I thought, and there I remained. It was very cold, and I froze my feet and hands. I then felt that the devils were burning off my feet, and I shrieked for liquor. I looked down and saw a bottle at my feet, but when I reached down to get it a lion threw his claws over it, and warned me with a fierce growl not to touch it. The snow melted, the season changed, and I was standing in mud and mire up to my neck. Ropes were tied around me, and horses were hitched to them to drag me from the deeps, but in trying to draw me out the ropes would snap asunder and I was left imbedded in the clay. They could not move me, because Christ had commanded me to stand there. A little while before the break of day the Savior appeared and told me to go. I started to run, but when I got alongside the old depot there burst from it the combined screams of millions of incarnate devils. I can hear in fancy still the avalanche of voices which rolled from those lost myriads. I ran into the first house to which I came. Its saw at a glance what was the nature of my terrible trouble, but he had no power to help me. I beheld the face of a black fiend grinning on me through a window. In the center of his forehead was an enormous and fiery eye, and about his sinister mouth the grin which I at first saw became demoniacal. He called the fiends, and I heard them come as a rushing tornado, and surround the house. Everything I attempted to do was anticipated by them. If I thought of moving my hand I heard them say, "Look! he is going to lift his hand." No matter what I did or thought of doing, they cursed me.

When daylight at last came - and oh, what an age of dying agony lay behind it in the vast hollow darkness of the night! - the horrid objects disappeared, but the voices remained and talked with me all day. You who read, imagine yourselves alone in a room, or walking deserted streets, with voices articulating words to you with as clear distinctness as words were ever spoken to you. Many of the voices were those of friends and acquaintances whom I knew to be in their graves, and yet they - their voices - were conversing with, or talking to me, during the whole of that long, long, terrible day. I was tortured with fears and a dread of something infinitely horrible. I went to my office - the voices were there! I stepped to the window, and on the street were men congregating in front of the building. I could hear their voices, and they were all talking of hanging me. I had committed an appalling crime, they said. I knew not where to go or whither to fly. Now and then I could hear strains of music. The dreaded night came on, and with it the fiends returned. In the excitement of breaking from my office, I forgot to put on my overcoat. The moment I got on the street the freezing wind drove me back, but hundreds of voices gathered around me and threatened me with death if I entered the door again. I went away followed by them, and wandered in a thin coat up and down the streets, and through the woods all night. The wonder was that I did not freeze to death. I could hear crowds of excited people at the court house discussing me, I thought. When I started to go there, every door and window of the building flew open and fiery devils darted out and cursed me away. All the time I was dying for whisky, but the saloon keepers would not give me a drop. They saw and understood what was the matter with me, and refused to finish the work begun in their dens. I started at last in the direction of home. Just outside of the town a man by my side showed me a bottle of whisky. I was dying for it, and begged him for at least one swallow. He opened the bottle and held it to my lips, and I saw that the bottle was full of blood. Again and again did he deceive me. Exhausted at last, I sank down in the snow and begged for death to come and end my life, but instead, a company of citizens of Rushville, whom I knew, gathered around me and a glass of whisky was handed to me. I saw that everyone present held a similar glass in his hand, which, at a given word, was raised to the mouth. I hastened to drink, but while they drained their glasses, I could not get a drop from mine. I looked more closely at the glass and discovered that there were two thicknesses to it, and that the liquor was contained between them. I studied how I could break the glass and not spill the whisky, and begged and plead with the men to have mercy on me. I got out into the woods four or five miles from Rushville, and wandered about in the snow, but all around and above me were the universal and eternal voices threatening me. A thousand visions came and went; a thousand tortures consumed me; a thousand hopes sustained me.

I quit the woods pursued by winged and cloven-footed fiends, and ran to the house of Andy Hinchman. He received and gave me shelter until morning, when he carried me back home in his buggy. I had no more than got into his house when it was surrounded by my tormentors. They raised the windows and commenced throwing lassos at me, in order, as they said, to catch me and drag me out that they might kill me. I sat up in my chair until daylight, fighting them off with both hands. All these terrible torments were, I repeat, realities, intensified over the ordinary realities of life a hundred fold. I had wandered to and fro, as I have described, but the people, the angels and the devils were alike the phantasmagoria of my diseased mind. For one week after the night last mentioned, I had no use of either arm. I had so frozen my feet that I could not put on my boots. Mr. Hinchman kindly loaned me a pair that I succeeded, although with great pain, in drawing on, for they were three sizes larger than I was in the habit of wearing. The devils were still with me, but I had moments of reason when I could banish them from my mind. On our way to town they rode on top of the buggy and clung to the spokes of the wheels, and whirled over and over with dizzy revolutions. How they fought, and cursed, and shrieked! When I got to my room it was the same, and for days I was surrounded the greater part of the time with demons as numberless as those seen in the fancy of the mighty poet of a Lost Paradise marshaled under the infernal ensign of Lucifer on the fiery and blazing plains of hell! For more than one month after the madness left me I was afraid to sleep in a room alone, and the least sound would fill me with fear. I ran when none pursued, and hid when no one was in search of me. My sleep was fitful and full of terrible dreams, and my days were days of unrest and anguish unspeakable.

# CHAPTER VIII

*Wretchedness and degradation - Clothes, credit, and reputation all lost - The prodigal's return to his father's house - Familiar scenes - The beauty of nature - My lack of feeling - A wild horse - I ride him to Raleigh and get drunk - A mixture of vile poison - My ride and fall - The broken stirrups - My father's search - I get home once more - Depart the same day on the wild horse - A week at Lewisville - Sick - Yearnings for sympathy.*

My condition now grew worse from day to day. I descended step by step to the lowest depths of wretchedness and degradation. Often my only sleeping-place was the pavement, or a stairway, or a hall leading to some office. I lost my clothes, pawning most of them to the rum-sellers, until I was unfit to be seen, so few and dirty and ragged were the garments which I could still call my own. In ten years I have lost, given away, and pawned over fifty suits of clothes. Within the three years just past I have had six overcoats that went the way of my reputation and peace of mind.

I left Rushville at the time of which I am writing, but not until it was out of my power to either buy or beg a drop of liquor - not until my reputation was destroyed and everything else that a true man would prize - and then, like the prodigal who had wallowed with swine, I returned to my father's house - the home of my childhood, around which lay the scenes which were imprinted on my mind with ineffaceable colors. But I had destroyed the sense which should have made them comforting to me. I have no doubt that nature is beautiful -

that there are fine souls to whom she is a glorious book, on whose divine pages they learn wisdom and find the highest and most exalting charms. But I, alas, am dead to her subtle and sacred influences. However, I might have been benefited by my stay at home, had it been difficult for me to find that which my appetite still craved; but it was not so. Falmouth and Raleigh and Lewisville were still within easy reach, and not only at these, but at many other places could liquor be procured, and I got it. The curse was on me. My condition became such that it was unsafe to send me from home on any business. I can recall times when I left horses hitched to the plow or wagon and went on a spree, forgetting all about them, for weeks. I had left home firm in the resolve to not touch a drop of liquor under any circumstances, and so thoroughly did I believe that I would not, that I would have staked my soul on a wager that I would keep sober. But the sight of a saloon, or of some person with whom I had been on a drunk, or even an empty beer keg, would rouse my appetite to such an extent that I gave up all thoughts of sobriety and wanted to get drunk. I always allowed myself to be deceived with the idea that I would only get on a moderate drunk this time, and then quit forever. But the first drink was sure to be followed by a hundred or a thousand more.

Once while in a state of beastly intoxication at Rushville, my father came for me and took me home in a wagon, and for two weeks I scarcely stirred outside of the house. But the house which should have been a paradise to me was made a prison by reason of my desires for the hell-created liberty of entering saloons and associating with men as reckless as myself. I became morose, nervous, and uneasy. I took a horseback ride one morning and would not admit to myself that I cared less for the ride than to feel that I could go where I could get liquor. I did not want to drink, but like the moth which returns by some fatal charm again and again to the flames which eventually consume it, I could not resist the temptation to go where I could lay my hands on the curse. There was on the farm, among the horses, one that was unusually wild, which had hitherto thrown every person that mounted it. The only way it could be managed at all was with a rough curb-bitted bridle, and even then each rein had to be drawn hard. If there was any one thing on which I prided myself at that time it was my proficiency in riding horses. I determined on mastering this horse, and early one morning I mounted his back. I got along without a great amount of difficulty in keeping my seat until I got to Raleigh. Here I dismounted and sat in the corner groceries for an hour or more, talking to acquaintances. Finally, like the dog returning to his vomit, I crossed the street and went into a saloon. Had the door opened into the vermilion lake of fire I would have passed through it if I had been sure of getting a drink, so sudden and uncontrollable was the appetite awakened. Only a few minutes before I had with religious solemnity assured two young men who were keeping a dry goods store there that I had quit drinking forever. To test me, I suppose, one of them had said to me that he had some excellent old whisky, and wanted me to try a little of it, and offered me the jug. I carried it to my mouth, and took a swallow. It was a villainous compound of whisky, alcohol and drugs of various kinds, which he sold in quart bottles under the name of some sort of bitters which were warranted to cure every disease: and I will add that I believe to this day that they would do what he said they would, for I do not think any human being, bird, or beast, unless there is another Quilp living, could drink two bottles of it in that number of days and not be beyond the need of further attention than that required to prepare him for burial. It was the sight of the jug and the taste of the poison slop which it contained that aroused my appetite and scattered my resolves to the tempest. Once in the saloon I drank without regard to consequences, and without caring whether the horse I rode was as jaded and tame as Don Quixote's ill-favored but famous steed, or as wild and unmanageable as the steed to which the ill-starred Mazeppa was lashed. I did not stop to consider that a clear head and steady hand were necessary to guide that horse and protect my life, which would be endangered the moment I again mounted my horse. Ordinarily I would have gone away and left the horse to care for itself, but I remembered the character of the horse, and with a drunken maniac's perversity of feeling I would not abandon it. I designed getting only so drunk, and then I would show the folks what a young man could really do. On leaving the saloon I returned to the jug, which contained the mixture described, and which would have called up apparitions on the blasted heath that would have not only startled the ambitious thane, but frightened the witches themselves out of their senses.

I took one full drink - what is called in the vernacular of the bar room a "square" drink - from the jug, and that, uniting with the saloon slop, made me a howling maniac. I have forgotten to mention that I got a quart of as raw and mean whisky in the saloon as was ever sold for the sum which I gave for it - fifty cents. It was about nine o'clock at night when I bethought me of the horse which I had sworn to ride home that evening. I untied the beast with some difficulty, and led him to a mounting block. I got on the block, and, after putting my foot securely in the stirrup, fell into the saddle, I was too drunk to think further, and so permitted the horse to take whatever course suited it best. It took the road toward home, but not as quietly as a butterfly would have started. He flew with furious speed, onward through the night, bearing me as if I had only been a feather. I did not, for I could not, attempt to control him. It was a race with death, and the chances were in death's favor long before we reached the home stretch. Possibly I might have ridden safely home had the road been a straight one, but it was not, and, on making a short turn, I was thrown from the saddle, but my feet were securely fastened in the stirrups, and so I was dragged onward by the animal, which did not pause in its mad career, but rather sped forward more wildly than ever. I was dragged thus over a quarter of a mile, and would undoubtedly have been killed had not one and then the other stirrup broken. I lay with my feet in the detached stirrups until near morning, wholly unconscious and dead, I presume, to all appearances. It was quite a while after I came to my senses before I could realize what had happened, who, and what, and where I was, and then my knowledge was too vague to enable me to determine anything definitely. I crawled to a house which was near by, fortunately, and remained there during the morning. I was badly, but not dangerously, injured. The skin was torn from one side of my face, and three of my fingers were disjointed. I was bruised all over, and cut slightly in several places. How I escaped death is a miracle, but escape it I did. The horse went on home and was found early in the morning, with the stirrup leathers dangling from the saddle. When the family saw the horse they at once were of the opinion that I had been killed, and my father took the road to Raleigh immediately, thinking to find my dead body on the way. Fearing that they would discover the horse and be frightened about me, I started home, and had not gone far when I met my father. As soon as he saw me walking in the road, he burst into tears. I did not dare look as he rode up to me, but continued walking, and he rode slowly past me. I could hear his sobs, but was too much overcome with shame to speak. I walked on toward home as fast as I could, and my heart-broken but happy father followed slowly in my rear. When I got within sight of the house my sister saw me and ran to meet me, crying: "Oh, we thought you were killed this time - I was sure you were killed. It is so dreadful to think of!" etc. She was crying and laughing in a breath. My feelings were such as words can not describe. I wanted the earth to open and swallow me up. I suffered a thousand deaths. This is only one of a hundred similar debauches, each more deplorable and humiliating in its consequences than the last.

At times, as the waters of the awful sea called the Past dash over me, I almost die of strangulation. I pant and gasp for breath, and shudder and tremble in my terror. My spree on this occasion was not yet over; my appetite was burning and raging, and notwithstanding my almost miraculous escape from a drunken death, I watched my opportunity, like a man bent on self-destruction, and again mounted the same horse and started for Raleigh. But my father had preceded me, and given orders at the saloon and elsewhere that I should not be allowed more liquor. I was determined to satisfy my appetite, and with this purpose subjugating every other, I went on to Lewisville, where I remained for more than a week, drinking day and night. Finally one of my brothers, hearing of my whereabouts, came after me and took me home. I was so completely exhausted the moment that the liquor began to die out that I had to go to bed, and there I remained for some time. After such debauches the physical suffering is intense and great; but it is little in comparison with the tortures of the mind. After such a spree as the one just mentioned, it has generally been out of my power to sleep for a week or longer after getting sober. I have tossed for hours and nights upon a bed of remorse, and had hell with all its flames burning in my heart and brain. Often have I prayed for death, and as often, when I thought the final hour had come, have I shrunk back from the mysterious shadow in which flesh has no more motion. Often have I felt that I would lose my reason forever, but after a period of madness, nature would be merciful and restore me my lost senses. Often have I pressed my hands tightly over my mouth, fearing that I would scream, and as often would a low groan sound in my blistered throat, the pent up echo of a long maniacal wail. Often have I contemplated suicide, but as often has some benign power held back my desperate hand; once, indeed, I tried to force the gates of death by an attempt to take my own life, but, heaven be forever praised! I did not succeed, for the knife refused to cut as deep as I would have had it. I thought I would be justifiable in throwing off by any means such a load of horror and pain as I was weighed down with. Who would not escape from misery if he could? I argued. If the grave, self-sought, would hide every error, blot out every pang, and shield from every storm, why not seek it?

They have in certain lands of the tropics a game which the people are said to watch with absorbing interest. It is this: A scorpion is caught. With cruel eagerness the boys and girls of the street assemble and place the reptile on a board, surrounded with a rim of tow saturated with some inflammable spirit. This ignited, the torture of the scorpion begins. Maddened by the heat, the detested thing approaches the fiery barrier and attempts to find some passage of escape, but vain the endeavor! It retreats toward the center of the ring, and as the heat increases and it begins to writhe under it, the children cry out with pleasure - a cry in which, I fancy, there is a cadence of the sound which sends a thrill of delight through hell - the sound of exultation which rises from the tongues of bigots when the martyr's soul mounts upward from the flames in which his body is consumed. Again the scorpion attempts to escape, and again it is turned back by that impassable barrier of fire. The shouts of the children deepen. At last, finding that there is no way by which to fly, the hated thing retreats to the center of its flaming prison and stings itself to death. Then it is that the exultation of the crowd of cruel tormentors is most loudly expressed. But do not infer from what I have said that I look with favor on suicide under any circumstances. That I do not do, but I would have you look at society and some of its victims.

See what barriers of flame are often thrown around poor, despairing, miserable men! Listen to that indifference and condemnation, and this wail of agony! Can you wonder that the outcast abandons hope and plunges the knife into his heart? He is driven to madness, and feeling that all is lost, he commits an act which does indeed lose everything for him, for it bars the gates of heaven against him. Before he had nothing on earth; now he has nothing in paradise. Alas for those who triumph over the fall of a fellow creature. God have mercy on those who exult over the wretchedness of a victim of alcohol! Woe to those who ridicule his efforts to escape, and who mock him when he fails. Do they not help to shape for him the dagger of self-destruction? What ingredients of poison do they not mix with the fatal drink which deprives him of breath? With what threads do they strengthen the rope with which he hangs himself! Where should the most blame rest, where does it most rest in the eyes of God - with society which drives him forth a depraved and friendless creature? or with himself no longer accountable for his acts? O the agony of feeling that on the whole face of the earth there is not a face that will look upon you in kindness, nor a heart that will throb with compassion at sight of your misery! I know what this agony is, for in my darkest hours I have looked for pity and strained my ears to catch the tones of a kindly voice in vain. But let me hasten to say, lest I be misunderstood, that since I commenced to lecture, I have had the support and active help of thousands of the very best men and women in the land. I doubt that there was ever a man in calamity trying to escape from terrors worse than those of death who had more aid than has been extended to me. Could prayers and tears lift one out of misfortune and wretchedness I would long ago have stood above all the tribulations of my life. I desire to have every man and woman that has bestowed kindness on me, if only a word or look, know that I remember such kindness, and that I long to prove that it was not thrown away. Every day there rises before me numberless faces I have met from time to time, each beautiful with the love, sympathy, and pity which elevates the human into the divine. There are others, I regret to say, that pass before me with dark looks and scowls. I know them well, for they have sought to discourage and drag me down. Their tongues have been quick to condemn and free to vilify me. I seek no revenge on them. I forgive as wholly and freely as I hope to be forgiven. May God soften their tiger hearts and melt their hyena souls.

# CHAPTER IX

*The ever-recurring spell - Writing in the sand - Hartford City - In the ditch - Extricated - Fairly started - A telegram - My brother's death - Sober - A long night - Ride home - Palpitation of the heart - Bluffton - The inevitable - Delirium again - No friends, money, nor clothes - One hundred miles from home - I take a walk - Clinton county - Engage to teach a school - The lobbies of hell - Arrested - Flight to the country - Open school - A failure - Return home - The beginning of a terrible experience - Two months of uninterrupted drinking - Coatless, hatless, and bootless - The "Blue Goose" - The tremens - Inflammatory rheumatism - The torments of the damned - Walking on crutches - Drive to Rushville - Another drunk - Pawn my clothes - At Indianapolis - A cold bath - The consequence - Teaching school - Satisfaction given - The kindness of Daniel Baker and his wife - A paying practice at law.*

I was at all times unhappy, and hence I was always restless and discontented. I was continually striving for something that would at least give me contentment, but before I could establish myself in any thing the ever-recurring spell would seize me, and whatever confidence I had succeeded in gaining was swept away. I wrote in sand, and the incoming tide with a single dash annihilated the characters. During one of my uneasy wanderings I went to Hartford City, Indiana. Hartford "City," like all other cities In the land, has a full supply of saloons. With a view of advertising myself I had my friends announce on the second day after my arrival that I would deliver a political speech. This speech was listened to by an immense crowd, and heartily praised by the party whose principles I advocated. I was puffed up with the enthusiasm of the people, and repaired with some of the local leaders to a saloon to take a drink in honor of the occasion. The drink taken by me as usual wrought havoc. I wanted more, as I always do when I take one drink, and I got more. I got more than enough, too, as I always do. On the way home with a gentleman whom I knew, I fell into a ditch, but was extricated with difficulty, and finally carried to the house of a friend. My clothes were wet and covered with mud. After sleeping awhile I got up and stole from the house very much as a thief would have sneaked away. I was fairly started on another spree, and for three weeks I drank heavily and constantly. Sometime during the third week of my debauch I received a telegram stating that my brother was dead. The suddenness and terrible nature of the news caused me to become sober at once. It was just at twilight when I received the telegram, and there was no train until nine o'clock the next morning. That night seemed like an age to me. I never closed my eyes in sleep, but lay in my bed weak and terror-stricken, waiting for the morning. It came at last, for the longest night will end in day. I got on the train and sat down by a window. I was so weak and nervous that I could not hold a cup in my hand. But I wanted no more liquor. The terrible news of the previous day had frightened away all desire for drink. I had not ridden far when I was seized with palpitation of the heart. The sudden cessation from all stimulants had left my system in a condition to resist nothing, and when my heart lost its regular action, the chances were that I could not survive. All day I drew my breath with painful difficulty, and thought that each respiration would be the last. I raised the car window and put out my head so that the rushing air would strike my face, and this revived me. When I got home my brother was buried. I had left him a few days before in good health and proud in his strength. I returned to find him hidden forever from my sight by the remorseless grave. What I felt and suffered no one knew, nor can ever know. Every night for weeks I could see my brother in life, but the cold reality of death came back to me with the light of day. I was stunned and almost crazed by the blow, and yet there were not wanting persons who, incapable of a deep pang of sorrow, said that I did not care. Could they have been made to suffer for one night the agony which I endured for weeks they would learn to feel for the miseries of others, and at the same time have a knowledge of what sufferings the human heart is capable.

My next move was to Bluffton, Wells county, Indiana, where I arranged to go into the practice of the law. But here at Bluffton, as elsewhere, were the devil's recruiting offices - the saloons - and the first night after I reached the town I got drunk. I remained in Bluffton until I got over the debauch, which embraced a siege of the delirium tremens more horrible than that already described. When I came to myself, I determined that I would go home. I was without money; I had no friends in Bluffton, and but few clothes to my back, and it was over one hundred miles to my father's, but I started on foot and walked the whole way. I stayed quietly at home a few days, and then went to Howard and Clinton counties on business, which was to make some collections on notes for other parties. While in Clinton county I engaged to teach a district school, and in order to begin at the time specified by the trustees, I returned home to get ready. I started to return to Clinton county on Friday, so as to be there to open school on the following Monday. I got off the train at Indianapolis, and went into one of the numerous lobbies of hell near the depot. It was a week from that evening before I was sober enough to realize where I was, who I was, where I had come from, and whither I had started. I could hardly believe it possible that I had fallen again, but there was no doubt of the fact. I had been arrested and had pawned my trunk to get money to pay my fine. To this day I don't know why I was arrested, but for being drunk, I suppose. I fled from the city, and walked thirty miles into the country, where I borrowed enough money of a friend to redeem my trunk. I then started for my school. Notwithstanding I was one week behind, the trustees were still expecting me, and on Monday morning, one week later than the time appointed at first, I opened school. But I was so worn out and confused in my faculties that at noon I was forced to dismiss the school. I hurried from the house to a small village in the neighborhood and there I got more liquor. The next morning I left for home. Such a condition of affairs was lamentable and damnable, but I was powerless to make it better. I have often wondered what the people of that neighborhood thought when they found that I had taken a cargo of whisky and disappeared as mysteriously as I came. If the young idea shot forth at all during that season among the children of that district it was directed by other hands than mine. I never sent in a bill for the sixty-two and a half cents due me for that half day's work. If the good people of Clinton will consent to call the matter even, I will here and now relinquish every possible claim, right, or title to the aforesaid amount. They have probably long since forgotten the school which was not taught, and the pedagogue who did not teach. I arrived at home in course of time, and remained there a few days.

It was not long until my restless disposition drove me forth in search of some new adventure, and now comes the brief and imperfect recital of the most terrible experiences of my life. On the first of July I began to drink, and it was not until the first of September that I quit. During this time I went to Cincinnati twice, once to Kentucky, and twice to Lafayette. I traveled nearly all the time, and much of the time I was in an unconscious state. I started from home with two suits of clothes which I pawned for whisky after my money was all gone. I arrived at Knightstown one day without coat, vest or hat. I was also barefooted. A friend supplied me with these necessary articles, and as soon as I put them on I went to a saloon kept by Peter Stoff, and there I staid four days without venturing out on the street. As soon as I was able, I took up my journey homeward. When I got to Raleigh I was so completely worn out that I dropped down in a shoe shop and saloon, both of which were in the same compartment of a building. That night I took the tremens. The next day my father came after me in a spring wagon, and hauled me home. For the most part, during the two months of which I speak, I had slept out doors, without even a dog for company, and I contracted slight cold and fever, which terminated in an attack of inflammatory rheumatism in my left knee. The rheumatism came on in an instant, and without any previous warning. The first intimation I had of it was a keen pain, such as I imagine would follow a knife if thrust through the centre of the knee. When the doctor reached the house my knee had swollen enormously. I was burning up with a violent fever, and was wild with delirium. He at once blistered a hole in each side of my knee, and applied sedatives. My suffering was literally that of the damned. I lay upon my back for days and nights on a small lounge, without sleeping a wink, so great was my suffering. For forty-eight hours my eyes were rolled upward and backward in my head in a set and terrible rigidity. In my delirium, I thought my room was overran by rats. I tried to fight them off as they came toward me, but when I thought they were gone I could detect them stealing under my lounge, and presently they would be gnawing at my knee, and every time one of them touched me, a thrill of unearthly horror shot through me. They tore off pieces of my flesh, and I could see these pieces fall from their bloody jaws. No pen could describe my sickening and revolting sensations of horror and agony. For sixty days did I lie upon my back on that couch, unable to turn on either side, or move in any way, without suffering a thousand deaths. I experienced as much pain as ever was felt by any mortal being, and it is still a wonder to me how I survived. I was, on more than one occasion, believed to be dead by my friends, and they wrapped me in the winding sheet. Even then I was conscious of what they were doing, and yet I was unable to move a muscle, or speak, or groan. A horrible fear came over me that they would bury me alive. I seemed to die at the thought, but, had mountains been heaped upon me, it would have been as easy for me to show that I was not dead. But I would gradually regain the power of articulation, and then again would hope rise in the hearts of those who were watching. At last, but slowly, I recovered sufficiently to be able to leave my room. I procured a pair of crutches, and by their aid I could go about the house. Next I went out riding in a buggy, and after a time got so that I could walk without difficulty, though not without my crutches, for I did not yet dare to bear weight on my afflicted knee.

One day I went to Rushville, and - O, curse of curses! - gave way to my appetite. The moment the whisky began to affect me, I forgot that I had crutches, and set my lame leg down with my whole weight upon it. The sudden and agonizing pain caused me to give a scream, and yet I repeated the step a number of times. But the insufferable pain caused me to return home.

It was now winter. The Legislature was in session at Indianapolis, and I was promised a position, and, with this end in view, packed my trunk and bid good-by to the folks at home. At Shelbyville, at which place I had a little business to attend to, I took a drink. Just how and why I took it has been already told, for the same cause always influenced me. The same result followed, and at Indianapolis I kept up the debauch until I had traded a suit of clothes worth sixty dollars for one worth, at a liberal estimate, about sixty-five cents. I even pawned my crutches, which I still used and still needed. One day I went to a bath-room, and after remaining in the bath for half an hour, with the water just as warm as I could bear it, I resolved to change the programme, and, without further reflection, I turned off the warm and turned on water as cold as ice could make it. It almost caused my death. In an instant every pore of my body was closed, and I was as numb as one would be if frozen. Even my sight was destroyed for a few minutes, but I contrived to get out of the bath and put on my rags. I found my way, with some difficulty, to the Union Depot, and boarded a train, but I did not notice that it was not the train I wanted to travel on until it was too late for me to correct the mistake. I went to Zionsville, and lay there three days under the charge of two physicians. I then started again to go home, expecting to die at any moment. At last I reached Falmouth, and was carried to my father's, where I passed two weeks in suffering only equaled by that which I had already borne.

On again recovering my health, I began to look about for

something to do, and hearing of a vacant school east of Falmouth, and about four miles from my father's, I made application and was employed to teach it. It is with pride (which, after the record of so many failures, I trust will readily be pardoned) that I chronicle the fact that from the beginning to the end of the term I never tasted liquor. I look back to those months as the happiest of my life. I did what is seldom done, for in addition to keeping sober (which I believe most teachers do without an effort), I gave complete satisfaction to every parent, and pleased and made friends with every scholar (a thing, I believe, that most teachers do not do). Very bright and vivid in memory are those days, made more radiant by contrast with the darkness and degradation which lie before and after them. As I dwell upon them a ray of their calm light steals into my soul, and the faces of my loved scholars come out of the intervening darkness and smile upon me, until, for a brief moment, I forget my barred window, the mad-house, and my desolation, and fancy that I am again with them. I boarded with Daniel Baker, and can never forget his own and his good wife's kindness.

At the close of my school I was in better health and spirits than I had ever before been. I began to feel that there was still a chance for me to redeem the losses of the past, and I can not describe how happy the thought made me. I again began the practice of law, and for six months I devoted myself to my duties. I had a large and paying practice, and not once but often was I engaged in cases where my fees amounted to from fifty to one hundred dollars, and once I received two hundred and fifty dollars. I will further say that my clients felt that they were paying me little enough in each case, considering the service I rendered them. But during the latter part of the time I suffered much from low spirits and nervousness, and my desire for whisky almost drove me wild at times. I fought this appetite again and again with desperate determination, and how the contest would have finally ended I can not say had I not been taken down sick. The physician who was sent for prescribed some brandy, and on his second visit he brought half of a pint of it, to be taken with other medicine in doses of one tablespoonful at intervals of two hours. I followed his directions with care, so far as the first dose was concerned, but if the reader supposes that I waited two hours for another tablespoonful of that brandy he does my appetite gross injustice. Neither would I have him suppose that I confined the second dose to a tablespoon. I waited until my friends withdrew, making some excuse about wanting to be alone in order to get them to go out at once, and then I got out of bed and swallowed the remainder of that brandy at a gulp. A desperate and uncontrollable desire for the poison had possession of me, and beneath it my resolutions were crushed and my will helplessly manacled. I slipped out of the room at the first opportunity, and managed to get a buggy in which I drove off to Falmouth where I immediately bought a quart of whisky. This I drank in an incredibly short space of time, and after that - after that - well, you can imagine what took place after that. Would to God that I could erase the recollection of it from my mind! Days and weeks of drunkenness; days and weeks of degradation; money spent; clothes pawned and lost; business neglected; friends alienated; and peace and happiness annihilated by the fell, merciless, hell-born fiend - Alcohol! So much for a half pint of brandy prescribed by an able physician. The vilest and most deadly poison could scarcely have been worse. Perhaps I was to blame - at least I have blamed myself - for not imploring the doctor in the name of everything holy not to prescribe any medicine containing a drop of intoxicating liquor. But I was sick and weak, and my appetite rose in its strength at mention of the word brandy, and when I would have spoken it palsied my tongue. I could not resist. The inevitable was upon me.

Down, down, down I went, lower and ever lower. Down, into the darkness of desperation! - down, into the gulf of ruin! - down, where Shame, and Sin, and Misery cry to fallen souls - "Stay! abide with us!" I felt now that all I had gained was lost, and that there was nothing more for me to hope for. The destroying devil had swept away everything. I was no longer a man. Behold me cowering before my race and begging the pitiful sum of ten cents with which to buy one more drink -

begging for it, moreover, as something far more precious than life. I resorted then, as many times since, to every means in order to get that which would, and yet would not, satisfy my insatiate thirst. No one is likely to contradict me when I say that I know of more ways to get whisky, when out of money and friends, (although no true friend would ever give me whisky, especially to start on) than any other living man, and I sincerely doubt if there is one among the dead who could give me any information on the subject. Had I as persistently applied myself to my profession, and resorted to half as many tricks and ways to gain my clients' cases, it would have been out of the range of probability for my opponents to ever defeat me. I might have had a practice which would have required the aid of a score or more partners. I understand very well that such statements as this are not likely to exalt me in the reader's estimation, but I started out to tell the truth, and I shall not shrink from the recital of anything that will prejudice my readers against the enemy that I hate. I could sacrifice my life itself, if thereby I might slay the monster.

# CHAPTER X

*The "Baxter Law" - Its injustice - Appetite is not controlled by legislation - Indictments - What they amount to - "Not guilty" - The Indianapolis police - The Rushville grand jury - Start home afoot - Fear - The coming head-light - A desire to end my miserable existence - "Now is the time" - A struggle in which life wins - Flight across the fields - Bathing in dew - Hiding from the officers - My condition - Prayer - My unimaginable sufferings - Advised to lecture - The time I began to lecture.*

It has been but a few years since the Legislature of Indiana passed what is known as the "Baxter Liquor Law." Among the provisions of that law was one which declared that "any person found drunk in a public place should be fined five dollars for every such offense, and be compelled to tell where he got his liquor." It was further declared that if the drunkard failed to pay his fine, etc., he should be imprisoned for a certain number of days or weeks. This had no effect on the drunkard, unless it was to make his condition worse. Appetite is a thing which can not be controlled by a law. It may be restrained through fear, so long as it is not stronger than a man's will, but where it controls and subordinates every other faculty it would be useless to try to eradicate or restrain it by legislation. When a man's appetite is stronger than he is, it will lead him, and if it demands liquor it will get it, no matter if five hundred Baxter laws threatened the drunkard. Man, powerless to resist, gives way to appetite; he gets drunk; he is poor and has no money to pay his fine; the court tells him to go to jail until an outraged law is vindicated. In the meantime the man has a wife and (it may be) children; they suffer for bread. The poor wife still clings to her husband and works like a slave to get money to pay his fine. She starves herself and children in order to buy his freedom. You will say: "The man had no business to get drunk." But that is not the point. He needs something very different from a Baxter law to save him from the power of his appetite. Besides, the law is unjust. The rich man may get just as drunk as the poor man, and may be fined the same, but what of that? Five dollars is a trifle to him, so he pays it and goes on his way, while his less fortunate brother is kicked into a loathsome cell. There never has been, never can, and never will be a law enacted that prevent men from drinking liquor, especially those in whom there is a dominant appetite for it. The idea of licensing men to sell liquor and punishing men for drinking it is monstrous. To be sure, they are not punished for drinking it in moderation, but no man can be moderate who has such an appetite as I have. Why license men to sell liquor, and then punish others for drinking it? What sort of sense or justice is there in it, anyhow? There is a double punishment for the drunkard, and none for the liquor-seller. The sufferings consequent on drinking are extreme, and no punishment that the law can inflict will prevent the drunkard from indulging in strong drink if his own far greater and self-inflicted punishment is of no avail.

When a man has become a drunkard his punishment is complete. Think of law makers enacting and making it lawful, in consideration of a certain amount of money paid to the State, for dealers in liquors to sell that which carries darkness, crime, and desolation with it wherever it goes! The silver pieces received by Judas for betraying his master were honestly gotten gain compared with the blood money which the license law drops into the State's treasury - license money. What money can weigh in the balance and not be found wanting where starved and innocent children, broken-hearted mothers and sisters, and deserted, weeping wives are in the scale against it? Mothers, look on this law licensing this traffic, and then if you do not like it cease to bring forth children with human passions and appetites, and let only angels be born.

After the passage of this law making drunkenness an offense to be fined, I had all the law practice I could attend to in keeping myself out of its meshes and penalties. It kept me busy to avoid imprisonment - for I was drunk nearly all the time. I was indicted twenty-two times. But it is fair to say that in a majority of cases these indictments were found by men in sympathy with me, and whose chief object in having me arrested was to punish the men who sold me liquor. Another mistake! It is next to impossible to get a drunkard to tell where he got his liquor. Half the time he himself does not know where he got it. I never indicted a saloon keeper in my life. The sale of liquor has been legalized, and so long as that is the case I would blame no man for refusing to tell where he got his liquor. A law that permits an appetite for whisky to be formed, and then punishes its victim after money, health, and reputation are all gone, is a barbarous injustice. Instead of making a law that liquor shall not be sold to drunkards, better enact a law that it shall be sold only to drunkards. Then when the present generation of drunkards has passed away, there will be no more. I succeeded in escaping from the penalty of the indictments found against me. I plead, in most instances, my own case, and once or twice, when so drunk that I could not stand up without a chair to support me, I succeeded by resorting to some of the many tricks known to the legal fraternity, in wringing from the jury a verdict of "not guilty."

But all this was anything but amusing. I have never made my sides sore laughing about it. The memory of it does not wreath my face in smiles. It is madness to think of it. I lived in a state of perpetual dread. When in Indianapolis the sight of the police filled me with fear. And here a word concerning the Indianapolis police. There are, doubtless, in the force some strictly honorable, true, and kind-hearted men - and these deserve all praise. But, if accounts speak true, there are others who are more deserving the lash of correction than many whom they so brutally arrest. Need they be told that they have no right to kick, or jerk, or otherwise abuse an unresisting victim? Are they aware of the fact that the fallen are still human, and that, as guardians of the peace, they are bound to yet be merciful while discharging their duties? I have heard of more than one instance where men, and even women, were treated on and before arriving at the station house as no decent man would treat a dog. Such policemen are decidedly more interested in the extra pay they get on each arrest than in serving the best interests of the community. Many a poor man has been arrested when slightly intoxicated, and driven to desperation by the brutality of the police, that, under charitable and kind treatment, would have been saved. And I wish to ask a civilized and Christian people, if it is just the thing to take a man afflicted with the terrible disease of drunkenness, and thrust him into a loathsome, dirty cell? Would it not be not only more human, but also more in accord with the spirit of our intelligent and liberal age, to convey him to a hospital? I leave the discussion of this subject to other and abler hands.

At one time the grand jury at Rushville met and found a number of indictments against me. I was drunk at the time, but by some means learned that an officer had a writ to arrest me. I started at once to go to my father's. I was without means to get a conveyance, and so I started afoot out the Jeffersonville railroad. I had then been drunk about one month, and was bordering on delirium tremens. After walking a mile or more, my boot rubbed my foot so that I drew it off and walked on barefooted. My feelings can not be imagined. Fear and terror froze my blood. The night came on dark and dismal, and a flood of bitter, wretched thoughts swept over me, crushing me to the earth. Before me in the distance appeared the head-light of an engine. It seemed to look at me like a demon's eye, and beckon me on to destruction. I heard voices which whispered in my ears - "now is the time." A shudder crept over me. Should I end my miserable existence? I knew that a train of cars was coming. I could lie down on the track, and no one would ever know but I had been accidentally killed. Then I thought of my father, and brothers, and sisters, and as a glimpse of their suffering entered my mind, I felt myself held back. A great struggle went on between life and death. It ended in favor of life, and I fled from the railroad. I soon lost my way and wandered blindly over the fields and through the woods all that night. I was perishing for liquor when daylight came. In order to assuage my burning appetite I climbed over a fence, and, picking up a dirty, rusty wash-pan which had been thrown away, I drank a quart of water which I dipped from a horse-trough. My skin was dry and parched, and my blood was in a blaze. When I came to grassy plots I lay down and bathed my face in the cold dew, and also bared my arms and moistened them in the cool, damp grass.

When the sun came up over the eastern tree-tops I found that I was about ten miles from Rushville. After stumbling on for some time longer I found my way to Henry Lord's, a farmer with whom I was acquainted. He gave me a room in which I lay hidden from the officers for two days and nights. From this place I went to my father's, and although the officers came there two or three times, I escaped arrest. It is impossible to give the reader the faintest idea of my condition. Without money, clothes, or friends, an outcast, hunted like a wild beast, I had only one thing left - my horrible appetite, at all times fierce and now maddening in the extreme. My hands trembled, my face was bloated, and my eyes were bloodshot. I had almost ceased to look like a human. Hope had flown from me, and I was in complete despair. I moved about over my father's farm like one walking in sleep, the veriest wretch on the face of the earth. My real condition not unfrequently pressed upon me until, in an agony of desperation, I would put my swollen hands over my worse than bloated face and groan aloud, while tears scalding hot streamed down over my fingers and arms. I staid at home a number of days. At first I had no thought of quitting drink. I was too crazed in mind to think clearly on any subject. After two or three days, I became very nervous for lack of my accustomed stimulants; then I got so restless that I could not sleep, and for nights together I scarcely closed my aching eyes. Long as the days seemed, the nights were longer still. At the end of two weeks I began to have a more clear or less muddied conception of my condition, and a faint hope came to me that I might yet conquer the appetite which was taking me through utter ruin of body, to the eternal death of body and soul. The reader must not think that I thought I could by my own strength save myself. I prayed often and fervently. However strange it may sound it is nevertheless true, that, notwithstanding the degraded life I have lived, I have covered it with prayer as with a garment, and with as sincere prayer, too, as ever rose from the lips of pain and sin. My unimaginable sufferings have impelled me to seek earnestly for an escape from the torments which go out beyond the grave. None can ever be made to realize how much pain and agony I experienced during these first weeks I spent at home and abstained from liquor, nor can any know how much I resisted. At that time I had not the least thought of lecturing. Many times, when getting over a spree, I had, in the presence of people, given expression to the agonies that were consuming me, and at such times I did not fail to pay my respects to alcohol in a way (the only way) it deserves. My friends advised me to lecture on temperance, and I now began to think of their words. Was it my duty to go forth and tell the world of the horrors of intemperance, and warn all people to rise against this great enemy? If so, I would gladly do it. I began to prepare a lecture. It would help me to pass away the time, if nothing more came of it. It has been nearly four years since I delivered that lecture. I will give a history of my first effort and succeeding ones, with what was said about me, in the next chapter.

## CHAPTER XI

*My first lecture - A cold and disagreeable evening - A fair audience - My success - Lecture at Fairview - The people turn out en masse - At Rushville - Dread of appearing before the audience - Hesitation - I go on the stage and am greeted with applause - My fright - I throw off my father's old coat and stand forth - Begin to speak, and soon warm to my subject - I make a lecture tour - Four hundred and seventy lectures in Indiana - Attitude of the press - The aid of the good - Opposition and falsehood - Unkind criticism - Tattle mongers - Ten months of sobriety - My fall - Attempt to commit suicide - Inflict an ugly but not dangerous wound on myself - Ask the sheriff to lock me in the jail - Renewed effort - The campaign of '74 - "Local option."*

I delivered my first lecture at Raleigh, the scene of many of my most disgraceful debauches and most lamentable misfortunes. The evening announced for my lecture was unpropitious. Late in the afternoon a cold, disagreeable rain set in, and lasted until after dark. The roads were muddy, and in places nearly impassable. I did not expect on reaching the hall, or school house, or church in which I was to speak, to find much of an audience, but I was agreeably disappointed; for while the house was by no means "packed," there was still a fair audience. Raleigh had turned out en masse, men, women and children. I suppose they were curious to hear what I had to say, and they heard it if I am not much in error. I was much embarrassed when I first began to speak - more so than I have ever been since, even when in the presence of thousands. I did the best I could, and the audience expressed very general satisfaction. I think some of my statements astounded them a trifle, but they soon recovered and listened with profound and respectful attention. My next appointment was at Fairview. Here, as at Raleigh, I had often been seen during some of my wild sprees, and here, as at Raleigh, the people came out in force to hear me. I improved on my first lecture, I think, and felt emboldened to make a more ambitious effort. I settled on Rushville as the next most desirable place to afflict, and made arrangements to deliver my lecture there. A number of the best young men in the town of the class that never used liquor, but who had always sympathized with me, went without my consent or knowledge to the ministers of the different churches, and had them announce that on the next Monday evening Luther Benson, "the reformed drunkard," would lecture in the Court House. I was nervous from the want of my accustomed stimulants, and the added dread of appearing before an audience before whose members I had so many times covered myself with shame, and in whose Court House - the very place in which I was to speak - I had been several times indicted for violations of the law, almost caused me to break my engagement. While still hesitating on what course to take, whether to go before the audience or go home and hang myself, the dreaded Monday evening came, and with it came my friends to escort me to the stage, which had been extemporized for me. I waited until the last moment before entering the room.

On making my appearance I was greeted with applause, but instead of reassuring me, it frightened me almost out of my wits. However, it was too late to retreat, and so making up my mind to die, if necessary, on the spot, or succeed, I hastily threw off my father's old and threadbare overcoat (I had none of my own) and stood forth in a full dress coat, which showed much ill treatment, and immediately began my lecture. As I warmed to my work, and got interested, I forgot my embarrassment and talked with ease and volubility. I did not fail, in proof of which I have only to add that on the following day I met Ben. L. Smith on the street, and on the strength of my lecture, he went my security for a respectable coat and pair of boots.

From Rushville I started on a lecture tour, taking in Dublin, Connersville, Cambridge City, Shelbyville, Knightstown, Newcastle, and other places. By degrees I widened the field of my lectures until it embraced the whole of Indiana and parts of many other States. In a little more than three years I have spoken publicly four hundred and seventy times in Indiana alone. From the very first I have been warmly and generously supported by the press. There have been exceptions in the case of a few papers, but they were only the exceptions. Since my first effort to reform, all good people have aided me. But from the very first I have had to fight opposition and falsehood. I have been accused of being drunk when I was sober, and outrageous falsehoods have been told about me when the truth would have been bad enough. After I had got fairly started to lecture I had always one object paramount, and that was to save myself from the drunkard's terrible fate and doom. After a short time men who drank would come to me and congratulate me, saying that I had opened their eyes, and that from that day forward they would drink no more liquor. Mothers, wives, and sisters, who had sons, husbands, and brothers that indulged in the fatal habit, came to me and encouraged me by telling me how much good I had done them. I began to feel a strong additional motive to lecture and save others. And here I wish to say that my efforts to save all men whom I met that were in danger (and all are in danger who touch liquor in any form) of the curse, have been the cause of much unkind criticism. People have said: "O, well, we don't believe Benson is in earnest. He don't seem to try very hard to quit drinking himself. He doesn't keep the right sort of company," and so on. This was the language of men who never drank. I have had drinking men by the score come to me with tears in their eyes, and beg to know if there was any escape from the curse. Since taking the lecture field I have paid out in actual money over a thousand dollars to aid men and families in trouble caused by the use of liquor. I have the first one yet to turn away when I had anything to give. I have more than once robbed myself to aid others. Oftentimes my labor and money have been thrown away, but I have the satisfaction of knowing that I did my duty. In some cases, thank heaven! I have cause to know that my efforts were not in rain.

For ten months from the time I quit drinking and began to lecture, I averaged one lecture a day. I lived on the work and its excitement, making it take, as far as possible, the place of alcohol. I learned too late that this was the very worst thing I could have done. I was all the time expending the very strength I so much needed for the restoration of my shattered system. For ten months, lacking two days, I fought my appetite for whisky day and night. I waged a continued, never-ceasing, never-ending battle, with what earnestness and desire to conquer the God to whom I so fervently prayed all that time alone knows, and he alone knows the agony of my conflicts. I dreamed that I was wildly drunk night after night, and I would rise from my bed in the morning more weary than when, tired and worn out from overwork, I sought rest. The horror of such dreams can be known only to those who have experienced them. The shock to my nervous system from a sudden and complete cessation of the use of all stimulating drinks was of itself a fearful thing to encounter. I was often so nervous that, for nights at a time, I got little or no sleep. The least noise would cause me to tremble with fear. I suffered all the while more than any can ever know, save those who have gone through the same hell. The manners and actions often induced by my sufferings and an abiding sense of my afflictions not infrequently militated against me. It has often been said: "He acts very strangely - must have been drinking." Again: "I believe he uses opium." These assertions may have been honestly made, but they were none the less utterly false. If people could only know just how much the drunkard suffers; how sad, lonesome, gloomy and wretched he feels while trying to resist the accursed appetite which is destroying him, they would never taunt him with doubts, nor go to him, as I have had men, and even women, come to me (I say "men and women," but they were neither men nor women, but libels on men and women), and say that this or that person had said that that or this person had heard some other person tell another person that he, she, or it believed that I, Luther Benson, had been drinking on such and such an occasion; or that some one told Mr. B., who told Miss X.T. that J.B. had said to Madam Z. that such and such a one had actually told T.Y. that O.M.U. had seen three men who had heard of four other men who said they could find two women who had overheard a man say that he had seen a man who had seen me with two men that had a bottle of something which he felt pretty sure was Robinson county whisky. Therefore B. was drunk!

These things had the effect on me that this account will probably have on the reader - they annoyed me exceedingly at times. At times the falsehoods were more malicious still, causing me many sleepless hours. At the end of ten months of complete sobriety, during which I never tasted any stimulant - ten months of constant struggle and determined effort - I fell. Alas, that I am compelled to write the sad words! I had broken down my strength; my mental and physical energies gave way, and my appetite had wrapped itself as a flaming fire about me, consuming me in its heat. I commenced drinking at Charlottsville, Henry county, and went from there to Knightstown on a Saturday evening. On the following Monday I went to Indianapolis drunk, and there got "dead drunk." My friends in Rushville, hearing of my misfortune, came after me and took me with them to that place, where I remained utterly oblivious until the next Sunday, when, by some means - I have no knowledge how - I got on an early train that was passing through Rushville, and went as far as Columbus, where I got off, and soon succeeded in getting a quart of liquor. Between the hour of my arrival at Columbus and night I drank three bottles of whisky.

That night I returned to Rushville, and while mad with liquor, made an attempt on my life by cutting my throat. Well for me that my knife was dull and did not penetrate to the jugular artery. The wound self-inflicted was an ugly but not dangerous one. I kept on drinking for a week or more, until I found that it was utterly out of my power to resist drinking so long as I remained in a place where I could see, or buy, or beg whisky. I finally went to the sheriff and asked him to lock me up in jail, which I finally persuaded him to do. Once in jail I tried in vain to get more liquor. I remained there until the fierce fires of my appetite smouldered once more, and then I was released. I lay in bed sick several days at this time, sick in mind, soul, and body. I felt that for me there was nothing left. I had descended to the lowest depths. I was forever ruined and undone. Many who had said that I would not or could not stop drinking seemed to be delighted over my terrible misfortune. The smile with which they would say, "I told you so!" was devilish and fiendish. But many friends gathered about me and cheered me with hope that by renewed effort I might rise again. Well and truly did a great English poet, Campbell, I believe, say: -

"Hope springs eternal in the human heart."

I determined once more that I would not give up, I would fight my tireless enemy while a breath of life or an atom of reason remained in my being.

It was now July, 1874. An exciting political campaign was coming off, the main issue was "local option." I took the side and became an advocate of local option, and until the election in October, averaged one speech per day, frequently traveling all night in order to meet my engagements. That campaign broke me down completely, and on the first of November I again yielded, after a prolonged and desperate struggle, to the powers of my sleepless and tireless adversary. So terrible were the consequences of this fall that in the hope of preventing others from ever indulging in the ruinous habit which led to it, I wrote out and published a full account of it under the title of "Luther Benson's Struggle for Life." Inasmuch as this book will be incomplete without it, I will embody that brochure in the next chapter, so that those who have never read it may now do so, if they desire.

# CHAPTER XII

*Struggle for life - A cry of warning - "Why don't you quit?" - Solitude, separation, banishment - No quarter asked - The rumseller - A risk no man should incur - The woman's temperance convention at Indianapolis - At Richmond - The bloated druggist - "Death and damnation" - At the Galt House - The three distinct properties of alcohol - Ten days in Cincinnati - The delirium tremens - My horrible sufferings - The stick that turned to a serpent - A world of devils - Flying in dread - I go to Connersville, Indiana - My condition grows worse - Hell, horrors, and torments - The horrid sights of a drunkard's madness.*

Depraved and wretched is he who has practiced vice so long that he curses it while he yet clings to it; who pursues it because he feels a terrible power driving him on toward it, but, reaching it, knows that it will gnaw his heart, and make him roll himself in the dust. Thus it has been, and thus it is, with me. The deep, surging waters have gone over me. But out of their awful, black depths, could I be heard, I would cry out to all who have just set a foot in the perilous flood. For I am not one of those who, if they themselves must die the death most terrible and appalling of all others, would drag or even persuade one other soul to accompany them. But as the oblivious waves are surging about me, and as I try to brave and buffet them, I would cry to others not to come to me. When but just gasping and throwing up my hand for the last time, it would not be to clutch, but, if possible, to push back to safety. Could the youth who has just begun to taste wine, and the young man his first drink - to whom it is as delicious as the opening scenes of a visionary life, or the entering into some newly-discovered paradise where scenes of undimmed glory burst upon his vision - but see the end of all that, and what comes after, by looking into my desolation, and be made to understand what a dark and dreary thing it is for a man to be made to feel that he is going over a precipice with his eyes wide open, with a will that has lost power to prevent it; could he see my hot, fevered cheeks, bloodshot eyes, bloated face, swollen fingers, bruised and wounded body; could he feel the body of the death out of which I cry hourly, with feebler and feebler outcry, to be delivered; could he know how a constant wail comes up and out from my bleeding heart, and begs and pleads with a great agony to be delivered from this awful demon, drink; could these truths but go home to the hearts and minds of the young men of the land; could they feel for but one single moment what I am compelled to live, and battle, and endure day in, and day out, until the days drag themselves into weeks that seem like months, and months that seem like years, striving all the time, a living, walking, talking death, and cares, pleasures, and joys, all gone, yet compelled to endure and live, or rather die, on; could every young man feel these things as I am compelled to feel and bear them, it seems to me that it would be enough to make them, while they yet have the power to do it, dash the sparkling damnation to the earth in all the pride of its mantling temptation.

At the very threshold of blooming manhood I found myself subject to all the disadvantages which mankind, if they reflected upon them, would hesitate to impose upon acknowledged guilt. In every human countenance I feared to find an enemy. I shrank from the vigilance of human eyes. I dared not open my heart to the best affections of our nature, for a drunkard is supposed to have no love. I was shut up within my own desolation - a deserted, solitary wretch in the midst of my species. I dared not look for the consolation of friendship, for a drunkard is always the subject of suspicion and distrust, and is not supposed to be possessed of those finer feelings that find men as friends. Thus, instead of identifying myself with the joys and sorrows of others, and exchanging the delicious gifts of confidential sympathy, I was compelled to shrink back and listen to the horrid words, You are a drunkard - words the very mention or thought of which has ten thousand times carried despair to my heart, and made me gasp and pant for breath. Thus it was at the very opening of life, and thus it ever has been, and thus it is to-day. I have struggled, and with streaming eyes tried to wrench the chains from my bruised and torn body. My weary and long-continued struggles led to no termination. Termination! No! The lapse of time, that cures all other things, but makes my case more desperate. For there is no rest for me. Whithersoever I remove myself, this detestable, hated, sleepless, never-tiring enemy is in my rear. What a dark, mysterious, unfeeling, unrelenting tyrant! Is it come to this? When Nero and Caligula swayed the Roman scepter, it was a fearful thing to offend the bloody rulers. The Empire had already spread itself from climate to climate, and from sea to sea. If their unhappy victim fled to the rising of the sun, where the luminary of day seems to us first to ascend from the waves of the ocean, the power of the tyrant was still behind him; if he withdrew to the west, to Hesperian darkness and the shores of barbarian Thule, still he was not safe from his gore-drenched foe. Rum! Whisky! Alcohol! Fiend! Monster! Devil! Art thou the offspring in whom the lineaments of these tyrants are faithfully preserved? Was the world, with all its climates, made in vain for thy helpless, unoffending victim?

To me the sun brings no return of day. Day after day rolls on, and my state is immutable. Existence is to me a scene of melancholy. Every moment is a moment of anguish, with a trembling fear that the coming period will bring a severer fate. We talk of the instruments of torture, but there is more torture in the lingering existence of a man that is in the iron clutches of a monster that has neither eyes, nor ears, nor bowels of compassion; a venomous enemy that can never be turned into a friend; a silent, sleepless foe, that shuts out from the light of day, and makes its victim the associate of those whom society has marked for her abhorrence; a slave loaded with fetters that no power can break; cut off from all that existence has to bestow; from all the high hopes so often conceived; from all the future excellence the soul so much desires to imagine. No language can do justice to the indignant and soul-sickening loathing that these ideas excite. A thousand times I have longed for death, and wished, with an expressible ardor, for an end to what I suffered. A thousand times I have meditated suicide, and ruminated in my soul upon the different means of escaping from my load of existence. A thousand times in wretched bitterness I have asked myself, What have I to do with life? I have seen and felt enough to make me regard it with detestation. Why should I wait the lingering process of an unfeeling tyrant that is slowly tearing me to pieces, and not dare so much as die but when and how the marble-hearted thing decrees? Still, some inexplicable suggestion withheld my hand, and caused me to cling with desperate fondness to this shadow of existence, its mysterious attractions, and its hopeless prospects - appetite, fiendish thirst, a burning, ever-crying demand for a poison that is death, and for which a man will give his body and soul as a sacrifice to whoever will satisfy his imperious cravings. Let this appetite entwine itself about a man, let it throw its iron arms about his bruised body, and he will curse the day he was born. But some one says, Why don't you quit? Just don't drink! In answer I would say, O God, give me poverty, shower upon me all the hardships of life, turn me a prey to the wild beasts of the desert, so I be never again the victim of rum. Suffer me to call life and the pursuit of life my own, free from the appetite for alcohol, and I am willing to hold them at the mercy of the elements, the hunger of beasts, or the revenge of cold-blooded men. All of these, rather than the poison of the accursed cup.

Solitude! separation! banishment! These are words often in the mouths of human beings; but few men except myself have been permitted to feel the full latitude of their meaning. The pride of philosophy has taught us to treat man as an individual. He is no such thing. He holds, necessarily, indispensably, a relation to his species. He is like those twin births that have two heads and four hands, but if you attempt to detach them from each other, they are inevitably subjected to a miserable and lingering destruction. If a man wants to conceive a lively idea of the regions of the damned, just let him get himself in that condition that he is alone with an enemy while he is surrounded by society and his friends - an enemy that is like what has been described as the eye of Omniscience pursuing the guilty sinner and darting a ray that awakens him to a new sensibility at the very moment that otherwise exhausted nature would lull him into a temporary oblivion of the reproaches of his conscience. No walls can hide me from the discernment of my hated foe. Everywhere his industry in unwearied, to create for me new distress. Never can I count upon an instant of security; never can I wrap myself in the shroud of oblivion. The minutes in which I do not actually perceive and feel my destroyer are contaminated and blasted with the certain expectation of speedy interference. Thus it has been, and thus it is to-day, and with every returning day.

Tyrants have trembled, surrounded by whole armies of their janizaries. Alcohol - venomous serpent! robber and reviler! - what should make thee inaccessible to my fury? I will unfold a tale! I will show thee to the world for what thou art, and all the men that read shall confess my truth! Whisky - abhorrer of nature, the curse of the human species! - the earth can only be freed from an insupportable burden by thy extermination! Rum - poisoner! destroyer! that spits venom all around, and leaves the ground infected with slime! Accursed poison-makers and poison-dispensers! - do you imagine that I am altogether passive; a mean worm, organized to feel sensations of pain, but having no emotion of resentment? Did you imagine that there was no danger in inflicting on me pains, however great; miseries, however direful? Do you believe me impotent, imbecile, and idiot-like, with no understanding to contrive my escape and thy ruin, and no energy to perpetrate it? I will tell the end of thy infernal works. The country, in justice, shall hear me. I would that I had the language of fire, that my words might glow, and burn, and drop like molten lava, that I might wipe you from the face of the earth, or persuade mankind to turn away and starve you to death. Think you that I would regret the ruin that had overwhelmed you? Too long I have been tender-hearted and forbearing. Whisky, whisky sellers and whisky makers, traffickers and dealers in tears, blood, sin, shame, and woe! - ten thousand times you have dipped your bloody talons in my blood. There is no evil you have scrupled to accumulate upon me! Neither will I be more scrupulous. You have shown me no mercy, and you shall receive none.

Let us look at the rumseller, that we may know what manner of man he is, and then ask if he deserves the pity, sympathy, or respect of society, or any part of it. Viewed considerately, in the light of their respective motives, the drunkard is an innocent and honorable man in comparison with the retailer of drinks. The one yields under the impulse - it may be the torture - of appetite; the other is a cool, mercenary speculator, thriving on the frailties and vices of others. He is a man selling for gain what he knows to be worthless and pernicious; good for none, dangerous for all, and deadly to many. He has looked in the face the sure consequences of his course, and if he can but make gain of it, is prepared to corrupt the souls, embitter the lives, and blast the prosperity of an indefinite number of his fellow-creatures. By the selling of his poisons he sees that with terrible certainty, along with the havoc of health, lives, homes, and souls of men, he can succeed in setting afloat a certain vast amount of property, and that as it is thrown to the winds, some small share of it will float within his grasp. He knows that if men remain virtuous and thrifty, if these homes around him continue peaceful and joyous, his craft can not prosper. The injured old mothers, the wives, and the sisters are found where rum is sold. Orphan children throng from hut and hovel, and lift their childish hands in supplication, asking at the hands of the guilty whisky sellers for those who rocked their cradles, and fed and loved them. The murderer, now sober and crushed, lifts his manacled hands, red with blood, and charges his ruin upon the men who crazed his brain with rum. The felon comes from his prison tomb, the pauper from his dark retreat, where the rumseller has driven him to seek an evening's rest and a pauper's grave. From ten thousand graves the sheeted dead stalk forth, and with eyeless sockets and bared teeth, grin most ghastly scorn at their destroyers. The lost float up in shadowy forms, and wail in whispered despair. Angels turn weeping away, and God, upon his throne, looks in anger, and hurls a woe upon the hand which "putteth a bottle to his neighbor's lips to make him drunken." To balance all this fearful array of mischief and woe, flowing directly from his work, the dealer in ardent spirits can bring nothing but the plea that appetite has been gratified. There are profits, to be sure. Death finds it the most liberal purveyor for his horrid banquet, and hell from beneath it is moved with delight at the fast-coming profits of the trade; and the seller also gets gain. Death, hell, and the rumseller - beyond this partnership none are profited. Go and shake their bloody hands, you who will! The time will be when deep down in hell these miserable, blood-stained wretches will pant for one drop of water, and curse the day and hour that they ever sold one drop of liquor.

The experience of ages proves that the use of intoxicating agents invariably tends to engender a burning appetite for more; and he who indulges in them shall do it at the peril of contracting a passionate and rabid thirst for them, which shall ultimately overmaster the will of his victim, and drag him, unresisting, to his ruin. No man can put himself under the influence of alcoholic stimulants without incurring the risk of this result. It may not be perceptible at once. It may be interrupted, and while the bonds are yet feeble he may escape. But let the habit go forward, the excitement be often repeated, and soon a deep-wrought physical effect will be produced; a headlong and almost delirious appetite, of the nature of a physical necessity, will have seized the whole man as with iron arms, and crushed from his heart the power of self-control.

My whole nature was almost constantly demanding and crying out for stimulants. During the period that I abstained from them, and for two weeks before I touched or tasted them the last time, my agony was unbearable. In my sleep I dreamed that I was drinking, and dreamed that I was drunk. Day by day my appetite grew fiercer and more unbearable, until in my misery I walked my floor hour after hour, unable to sleep, and feeling that if I lay down I should die. One night, about a week before I yielded, I walked my room until midnight, suffering the torments of hell. I felt that I was dying, and rushed out of my room and walked and ran across fields and through the woods, panting and gasping for breath. I felt that my head was bursting to pieces. My blood boiled, and hissed, and foamed through my veins. I could feel my heart throb and beat as though it would burst out of my body. At that time I would have torn the veins of my arms open, if I could have drawn whisky from them. When light came, I found that I had walked and run seven miles since leaving my room at midnight. All that day I was burning up for liquor. Had I been where I could lay my hands on it, a thousand times that day I would have drank though it steeped my soul in rivers of death.

In just this condition I went to Indianapolis to address the Woman's Temperance Convention. I felt that I would drop dead before I finished my speech. That night I did not sleep more than an hour, and that was a miserable hour of sleep, in which I dreamed that I was drunk. I woke up with a burning thirst, and sharp pains darting through my brain. The very least noise would send a new pang to my head, and when I attempted to walk, my own footsteps would jar upon my brain as though knives were driven through it. The next day and night I fought it like a tiger, but my thirst only increased, and then one gets tired at last of fighting an enemy all day, knowing that he must confront that same enemy the next day, and the next, for one can not live always on a strain, always in fear, and doubt, and dread. The next day I started for Richmond, where I had business, intending to go from there to Cincinnati and Covington, and thence East. I got to Richmond, haunted, every inch of the road, with an inexpressible longing for stimulants. When I got there, I knew that I was where I could get a little rest from my intense suffering, for I could get whisky. When the thought of what would be the result of touching it forced itself on my mind, my agony was so terrible that I could feel the sweat streaming down my face, and I could have wrung water from my hair.

If ever there was a man in ruins, a perfect spectacle of utter desolation, I was that man, as I stood in the depot at

Richmond, burning up for whisky. Had I been standing on red-hot embers my sufferings could not have been more intense. I feel that I can almost hear some one say, "Why did you not pray? just go and ask God to help you." I have been told to do that ten thousand times by good-meaning men and women, who do not know how to pray as I do, and never will until (which God forbid) they have suffered as I have. I did pray, and beg, and plead for mercy and help, but the heavens were solid brass and the earth hard iron, and God did not hear or heed my prayers. Talk about having the appetite for stimulants removed by prayer! That appetite is just as much the part of a man as his hand, heart, brain, or any other part of his body. Every one of God's laws are unchangeable and immutable. The day of miracles is over. When one of God's creatures violates his laws, he must pay the penalty; and I think it would be far better to educate the rising generation that there is no escape for them from the consequences of their acts, than to preach them into the belief that they may for years pursue a course of dissipation, violate every law of their being, and then by prayer have the chains of habit stricken off and be restored whole.

Then there is another class of individuals who have said to me, "When you get into that condition, when you feel that you must have liquor, why don't you just take a little in moderation?" Moderation! A drink of liquor is to my appetite what a red-hot coal of fire is to a keg of dry powder. You can just as easily shoot a ball from a cannon's mouth moderately, or fire off a magazine slowly, as I can drink liquor moderately. When I take one drink, if it is but a taste, I must have more, if I knew hell would burst out of the earth and engulf me the next instant. I am either perfectly sober, with no smell f of liquor about me, or I am very drunk. Some of those moderate drinkers, who are increasing their moderation a little every day, and also some pretended temperance people, who are always suspicious of others, because they are sneaking, cowardly, sly, deceitful and treacherous themselves, are constantly asking me if I do not drink a little all the time. And then they say I use morphine and opium. There is nothing that has made me more wretched, and done more to weaken and drag me down, than the continued accusation of doing something that it is just as impossible for me to do as it would be to live without breathing; that is, to take a drink of liquor without getting drunk. And if there is any one thing that will make me hate a man - loathe, abhor, and despise him - it is to have him accuse me of drinking or using any kind of stimulants regularly and moderately. I just want to say here, now, and for all time, that they who thus accuse me, lie in their teeth, mouth, throat, and away down deep in their dirty, cowardly, craven, black hearts.

I walked from the depot in Richmond - or, rather, almost ran - until I came to a drug store kept by a young man I have known for five or six years. He keeps nearly all drugs in barrels, well watered, and drinks them regularly, and, as he calls it, moderately. That is to say, he has not been sober for five years. Always full, bloated, imbecile, idiotic - has no idea of quiting himself, and would suffer as keenly as any brute is capable of suffering, at the thought of any one else who is in the habit of drinking becoming a sober man. When I went in, he was leaning back in a chair dozing, dreaming, drunk, or as drunk as that kind of a man generally gets. I asked him for whisky. He straightened up, and a more fiendish gleam of joy than lit up his brutal face never sat upon the hideous countenance of a fiend fresh from hell. He got up to get me the liquor, saying at the same time, "I will bet you five dollars you are drunk before night." I looked at him, saw the smile of joy, and the intense pleasure that my getting drunk was going to afford him. Suffering, choking, and almost bereft of reason, as I was, his look and act caused me to hesitate and wonder what manner of man it was that was so utterly base and heartless as to rejoice at the ruin of one whose continued prayer is to live and die sober. Then and there I prayed God to deliver me from such friends, and keep me from their accursed influence. Hell knows no blacker deformity than that which would drag a fellow-creature again to degradation. Satan was as much a friend of human happiness when he slimed into Eden. In my very youth, I made a resolve that I never would, knowingly, stand in the path of any man and a better life: that I would never do anything to prevent a man from leading a better life, and I have never broken that resolution. I gathered strength and courage enough, by a desperate effort, to get out of the store without drinking, and started in an opposite direction from where anything was kept to drink.

I had gone but a short distance, when there was no longer any enduring of the torture. I turned back and went into another drug store, and told the proprietor that I was sick, and asked him for whisky with some kind of medicine in it. The man who gave it was not to blame, for he knew nothing about me, nor the fiendish thirst with which I was possessed; and while he was not more than a minute getting the liquor for me, it seemed an age, and when I took the glass, I read "death" in it just as plainly as ever "death" was written upon the field of battle. I hesitated a moment, while something whispered, "Death!" I struggled, but could not let go of the glass. I felt the hot, scalding tears come in my eyes. I thought if I could only die - just drop dead; but I could not, yet I felt that I was dying ten thousand deaths all the time! I lifted the glass and drank death and damnation! I drank the red blood of butchery and the fiery beverage of hell! It glowed like hot lava in my blood, and burned upon my tongue's end. A smouldering fire was kindled. A wild glow shot through every vein, and within my stomach the demon was aroused to his strength. I had now but one thought, but one burning desire that was consuming me - that was for more drink! It crept to my fingers' ends, and out in a burning flush upon my cheek. Drink! - DRINK! I would have had it then if I had been compelled to go to hell for it! But I got it just one step this side the regions of the damned. I went to a saloon and commenced to pour it down, and continued until I was crazed. All power over my appetite was gone; I was oblivious to everything around me. I took the train for Cincinnati. I have a dim, shuddering remembrance of some parties at the depot trying to keep me from taking the cars. I don't know who they were, or what they said. I got to the city that night, and staid at the Galt House. I have no remembrance of anything from the time I left Richmond until I awoke next day about ten o'clock, with an aching head, swollen tongue, burnt, black, parched lips, and a thirst for whisky that was maddening. Death would have been kindness compared to what I suffered that morning.

And here let me ask the reader to indulge me for a while, that I may explain just the condition I was in, both physically and mentally. I know just how much charity I am to expect and receive from the corrupt wilderness of human society, for it is a rank and rotten soil, from which every shrub draws poison as it grows. All that in a happier field and purer air would expand into virtue and germinate into usefulness is converted into henbane and deadly nightshade. I know how hard it is to get human society to regard one's acts as other than his deliberate intentions. But of being a drunkard by choice, and because I have not cared for the consequences, I am innocent. I can say, and speak the truth, that there is not a person on earth less capable than myself of recklessly and purposely plunging himself into shame, suffering and sin. I will never believe that a man, conscious of innocence, can not make other men perceive that he has that thought. I have been miserable all my life. I have been harshly treated by mankind, in being accused of wickedly doing that which I abhor, and against which I have fought with every energy I possessed. The greatest aggravation of my life has been that I could not make mankind believe, or understand, my real and true condition. I can safely affirm that a blasted character, and the curses that have clung to my name, have all of them been slight misfortunes compared to this. I have for years endeavored to sustain myself by the sense of my integrity; but the voice of no man on earth echoed to the voice of my conscience. I called aloud, but there was none to answer; there was none that regarded. To me the whole world has been as unhearing as the tempest, and as cold as the iceberg. Sympathy, the magnetic virtue, the hidden essence of our life, was extinct. Nor has this been the whole sum of my misery. The food so essential to an intelligent existence, seemed perpetually renewing before me in its fairest colors, only the more effectually to elude my grasp and to attack my hunger. Ten thousand times I have been prompted to unfold the affections of my soul, only to be repelled with the greatest anguish, until my reflections continually center upon and within myself, where wretchedness and sorrow dwell, undisturbed by one ray of hope and light. It seems to me that any person but a fool would know that I had not purposely led the life of misery that has marked my steps for fifteen years. It would have been merciful in comparison, if I had planted a dagger in my heart, for I have suffered an anguish a thousand times worse than death. I would have had liquor that morning at Cincinnati if I had known that one single drink would have obliterated my body, soul, and spirit. I had no power to resist; and to prove that I was powerless, let us see what effect alcohol, in its physiological aspect, exerts.

Alcohol possesses three distinct properties, and consequently produces a threefold physiological effect.

1. It has a nervine property, by which it excites the nervous system inordinately, and exhilarates the brain.

2. It has a stimulating property, by which it inordinately excites the muscular motions, and the actions of the heart and blood-vessels.

3. It has a narcotic property. The operation of this property is to suspend the nervous energies, and soothe and stupefy the subject.

Now, any article possessing either one, or but two of these properties, without the other, is a simple and harmless thing compared with alcohol. It is only because alcohol possesses this combination of properties, by which it operates on various organs, and affects several functions in different ways at one and the same time, that its potency is so dreadful, and its influence so fascinating, when once the appetite is thoroughly depraved by its use. It excites and calms, it stimulates and prostrates, it disturbs and soothes, it energizes and exhausts, it exhilarates and stupefies simultaneously. Now, what rational man would ever pretend that in going through a long course of fever, when his nerves were impaired, his brain inflamed, his blood fermenting, and his strength reduced, that he would be able, through all the commotion and change of organism, to govern his tastes, control his morbid cravings, and regulate his words, thoughts and actions? Yet these same persons will accuse, blame, and curse the man who does not control his appetite for alcohol, while his stomach is inflamed, blood vitiated, brain hardened, nerves exhausted, senses perverted, and all his feelings changed by the accursed stuff with which he has been poisoning himself to death, piecemeal, for years, and which suddenly, and all at once, manifests its accumulated strength over him. In sixteen months I have fought a thousand battles, every one more fearful than the soldier faces upon the field of conflict, where it rains lead and hails shot and shell, and I have been victorious nine hundred and ninety-eight times. How many of these who blame me would have been more successful? A man does not come out of the flames of alcohol and heal himself in a day. It is struggle and conflict, and woe; but at last, and finally, it is glorious victory. And if my friends will not forsake me, I will promise them a victory over rum that shall be complete and entire. I have neither the heart nor the desire to attempt a description of my drunk at Cincinnati. Those who have never been in that condition could not understand it; and to those who have, it needs no description.

I was at the Galt House for about ten days, and during all that time I was as oblivious to all that was passing as if I had been dead and buried; I did not know day from night. I have no remembrance of eating anything during the whole time I was there. I only remember a burning thirst for whisky that seemed to be consuming me. The more I drank, the more I wanted. After the first four nights I could get no sleep, so I just staid up and drank all night, until, for the want of slumber, my whole body was torn with torment for long days and nights. I knew from former experience what was the awful ending! None who have ever even seen a victim cursed with delirium tremens will ever wish to look upon the like again. No human language can describe it; but its scenes burn in the eyeball so deeply that they never pass away. During the time, all the dread enginery of hell is planted in the victim's brain and he subject to its terrible torments. Most persons laugh at the idea of one having the tremens, and think it a sign of weakness. But there is more disgrace and shame for the man who can drink liquor to intoxication for ten years, and escape the drunkard's madness, than there is for the man who has had the tremens two or three times during that period. Tremens are brought about by the effects of the liquor upon the brain and nerves, and the less brain or nerves a man has the less liable he is to be a subject of the tremens. While in this situation the victim imagines that everything is real, and thinks and believes every object he sees actually exists. With this explanation, I will now proceed to tell what I have seen, felt, and heard, while in that condition.

I had felt the delirium tremens coming on for two or three days. I was just standing on the verge of a mighty precipice, unable to retrace my steps, and shuddering as I involuntarily leaned over and looked down into the vortex which my wild and heated imagination opened before me; and I could see the lost writhe, and hear them howl in their infernal orgies. The wail, the curse, and the awful and unearthly ha! ha! came fearfully up before me. I had got into that condition that not one drop of stimulants would remain on my stomach. I had been vomiting for more than forty-eight hours every drop that I drank. In that condition I went into a saloon and asked for a drink; and as I tremblingly poured it out, a snake shot its head up out of the liquor, and with swaying head, and glistening eye looking at me, licked out its forked tongue, and hissed in my face. I felt my blood run cold and curdle at my heart.

I left the glass untouched, and walked out on the street. By a terrible effort of my will, I, to some extent, shook off the terrible phantom. I felt that if I could get some stimulants to remain on my stomach I might escape the terrible torments that were gathering about me; and yet, at the very thought of touching the accursed stuff again, I could see the head of that snake, and could hear ten thousand hisses all around me, and feel it writhing and crawling through every vein of my body; while at the same time I was scorching and burning to death for more whisky. At that time I would have marched across a mine with a match touched to it; I would have walked before exploding cannons for more liquor. I went to another saloon, thinking I might get a drink to stay on my stomach, and steady my nerves, and give me strength to get home before I died; for I felt that this time there could be no escape from death. This time I was afraid to touch the bottle, and stood back, shaking and shuddering in every limb, while the murderer poured out the whisky; and again that liquor turned to snakes, and they crawled around the glass, and on the bar, and hissed, writhed, and squirmed. Then in one instant they all coiled about each other, and matted themselves into one snake, with a hundred heads; and from every head glittering eyes gleamed, and forked tongues hissed at me. I rushed from the saloon, and started, I did not know or care where, so that I might escape my tormentors. I had walked but a short distance, when a dog as large as a calf sprang up before me, and commenced to growl and snap at me. I picked up a stick about three feet long, thinking to defend myself; but just as soon as I took that stick in my hand, it turned to a snake. I could feel its slimy body writhe and squirm in my hands, and in trying to hold it to keep it from biting me, every finger-nail cut like a knife into the palm of my hand, and the blood streamed down over that stick, that to me was a living snake. Hell is a heaven compared to what I suffered at that time.

At last I dashed the cursed thing from me, and ran for my life. I got to some depot, I don't know what one, and took the cars. I didn't know or care where I went; at about ten miles above Cincinnati I left the cars. At times, for a little while, I could reason and understand my condition. I found, on looking around, that I was in a little town, where a young man lived who had been a college mate of mine. I went and told him my condition, and he did for me everything that one friend can do for another. But as night came on my tormentors returned in ten thousand hideous forms, and drove me raving mad. I went to a hotel, and there they persuaded me to lie down. Just as soon as I got to bed I reached my hand over, and it touched a cold, dead corpse. The room lighted up with a hundred bright lights, and that corpse, that now appeared to me like nothing that had ever been visible in human shape, opened its large, glassy, dead eyes, and stared me in the face. Then its whole face and form turned to a demon, and its red eyes glared at me, and its whole face was full of passion, fierceness and frenzy. I shrank back from the loathsome monster. On looking around, I beheld everything in my vision turn to a living devil. Chairs, stand, bed, and my very clothes, took shape and form, and lived; and every one of them cursed me. Then in one corner of my room, a form, larger and more hideous than all the others, appeared. Its look was that of a witch, or hag, or rather like descriptions that I had read of them. It marched right up to me, with a face and look that will haunt me to my grave. It began to talk to me, saying that it would thrust its fingers through my ribs, and drink my blood; then it would stick out its long, bony, skeleton-like fingers, that looked like sharp knives, and ha! ha! Then it said it would sit upon me and press me to hell; that it would roast me with brimstone, and dash my burnt entrails into my eyes. Saying this, it sprang at me, and, for what seemed to me an age, I fought the unearthly thing. At last it said, "Let me go!" and when it did, it glided to the door, and as it went out, gave me a fiendish look, and said, "I will soon be back, with all the legions of hell; I will be the death of you; you shall not be alive one hour." I left my room, and just as soon as I touched the street I stepped on a dead body. The whole pavement and street were filled; men, and women, and little children, lying with their pale faces turned up to heaven; some looked as though they were asleep; others had died in awful agony, and their faces wore horrid contortions; while some had their eyes burst from their heads. Every time I moved I stepped on a dead body, and it would come to life, and rear up in my face; and when I would step on a baby corpse it would wail in a plaintive, baby wail, and its dead mother would come to life and rush at me, while a thousand devils would curse me for stepping on the dead. I would tremble and beg, and try to find some place to put my feet; but the dead were in heaps, and covered the whole ground, so that I could neither walk nor stand without being on a corpse. If I stepped, it was on a dead body, and it would rise up and throw its arms about me, and curse me for trampling on it; and it was in this way that I put in that whole night.

When light dawned the horrible objects disappeared to some extent, and by a terrible effort I was able to control my mind, and reason on my condition. I was weak, nervous, and sick. I thought I would eat something, and try to gain a little strength. The very moment that I sat down to the breakfast table, every dish on that table turned to a living, moving, horrid object. The plates, cups, knives and forks became turtles, frogs, scorpions, and commenced to live and move toward me. I left the table without eating a bite. I went back to the city that day. I had but just got there when I wanted some whisky. I took a drink. During the day I drank as many as twenty glasses of liquor, and by evening I had got myself so steadied that I took the cars for home. I got as far as Connersville, where I remained during the balance of my drunk. I kept drinking for three or four days, and then commenced to vomit again. By this time I had got so weak that it was with the greatest effort that I could stand on my feet or walk one step. I felt the madness coming on again with tenfold fury. My terrible fear gave me more strength. I left the house, and started out on the road, and in an instant I was surrounded by what seemed a million of demons and devils; it seemed as though hell had opened up before me. The earth burst open under my feet, and hot, rolling flame was all around me. I could feel my hair and eyebrows scorch and burn; then in a moment everything would change. I could hear a thousand voices, all talking to me at the same time, and every one threatening me with some horrid death; then I would be surrounded with wild animals, fighting and tearing each other to pieces, and glaring at me, while devils told me they would tear me to pieces; then a tiger took my whole arm between his bloody jaws, and mashed and mangled it to pieces, and tore that arm from my shoulder; then some fiend, in the shape of an old hag, would come up and pour red-hot embers into the bleeding wound, from which my arm had been torn. When I screamed in agony, devils would laugh a horrid, devilish laugh.

I looked down and saw a jug of liquor at my feet, and when I reached down to get it I heard the click of a hundred pistols, and a grinning black devil threw his claws over the jug; then devils and witches boiled the whisky. I could see it on the fire, and hear it seethe and foam; then they danced around me, and said they had the liquor so hot that it would scald me to death; then they pried open my mouth, and poured it down my throat. I could feel my brain bursting out of my head, as that boiling liquor scalded and burned my tongue out of my mouth, and that tongue turned to a snake, and with forked tongue hissed at me.

The next thing I found myself standing on a railroad track; I could just see the headlight of the engine and hear the faint rumble of the cars, and when I tried to move off the track I found I was tied with a hundred ropes. It seemed to me there were a hundred devils up in the air, and each one had hold of a rope that was wound around my body in such a way that I could not move. The cars were coming closer and closer, faster and faster; the light of the engine looked like one horrid eye of fire; I could hear the rattle and rush of a thousand wheels; it was coming right on me with the rapidity of lightning. I could feel the beating of my heart, and my hair stood up and shook and shivered. The engine ran up to me and stopped, the hot smoke and steam choking and smothering me. The devils cursed and howled because the cars did not run over me; they said the next time there would come sure death; then they opened the doors of the engine, and threw in cats and dogs, men, women, and children. I could hear them scream as the hot flames wrapped themselves about them, until they would burst open; and that engine was red-hot. I could see the grin of skeleton demons, as, with a horrid curse, they motioned the engine to move back; and back, back it went, until I could just see a faint light; then, at the wild, cursing, screaming command of my tormentors, I could hear the cars coming again, faster and faster, closer and closer, and that engine ran at me just that way all night. It seemed just as real, and my sufferings were just as intense, as if it had been a reality. When morning came the devils left me, swearing that they would come back at night, and thus I was tortured all day with the dread of what was coming again at night. That day, as I was walking, hens and chickens would turn into little men and women; they were dressed up in bloody clothes; they would surround me, and pick my body full of holes; then they would pick my eyes out, and I could see my eyes dropping from their bloody bills.

When night came I went to my room. I could hear voices talking in all parts of the house. They would gather about me and whisper and talk about some way in which they would kill me; then the windows would be full of cats, and I could feel little kittens in my pockets; and when I walked I would step on kittens, and they would mew, and the old cats would howl and burst through the windows, and claw me to pieces. Then devils would take live, howling, squalling cats, and pound me with them until I was surrounded and walled in with dead cats. The more I suffered, and the harder I tried to escape, the more intense seemed their joy. The room would be full of every loathsome insect; they would crawl, fly, and buzz around me, stinging me in the face and eyes. Then the room would fill with rats and mice, and they would run all over me. Then ten thousand devilish forms would all rush at me. There were human forms of every size and shape. Some of them had the face and look of a demon, and from every part of the room their eyes glared at me; others had their throats gashed to the very spine, while every one of them accused me of being the cause of their misery. Then devils and men would rush at me and pin me to the wall of my room, by driving sharp, red-hot spikes through my body. I could see and feel the blood streaming from my wounds until my clothes were covered with it. Then they would take red-hot irons, and burn and scrape my flesh from my bones. They would pull and tear my teeth out, and dash them in my face. Then they would take sharp, crooked knife blades, and run them through my body, and tear me to pieces, and hold up before my eyes my bleeding, burned and quivering flesh, and it would turn to bloody, hissing snakes. Then I looked and could see my coffin and dead body. Then I came back to life again, and I heard voices under my head cursing me, and saying that they would bury me alive. At this the devils seized me, and I could feel myself flying through the air. At last they stopped, and I heard a heavy door open. They dragged me into what they told me was a vault, and, when I tried to escape, I found nothing but solid walls. The floor was stone, and slippery and slimy. I could hear rats and mice running over the floor. They would run up my sleeves and down my neck. In trying to escape from them I struck a coffin; it fell on the hard stone floor and burst open; then the room lighted up, and the skeleton from the burst coffin stood up before me, and a long, slimy snake crawled up and wrapped the skeleton to the very neck; and that horrid thing of bones, with a living snake coiled all about it, walked up to me and laid its bony fingers on my face. No language can give the least idea of the horrid sights and sufferings in the drunkard's madness.

# CHAPTER XIII

*Recovery - Trip to Maine - Lecturing in that State - Dr. Reynolds, the "Dare to do right" reformer - Return to Indianapolis - Lecturing – Newspaper extracts - The criticisms of the press - Private letters of encouragement - Friends dear to memory - Sacred names.*

After recovering from the debauch just described, which I did in the course of two or three days, I went East to the State of Maine, where I remained about three months, lecturing in all the principal cities, and in some of them a number of times. In Bangor, especially, I was warmly welcomed, and I spoke there as often as ten times, each time to a crowded house. Dr. Reynolds, the celebrated "Dare to do right" reformer, was at that time a resident of Bangor, and I had the honor to make his acquaintance. While in Bangor I made my headquarters at his office, and was much benefited and strengthened by coming in contact with him. Days and weeks passed, and I did not taste liquor, although at times, when depressed and tired from over-work, I found it difficult in the extreme to resist the cravings of my appetite.

I returned to Indianapolis in the spring of 1875. I remained in Indiana, lecturing almost daily, or nightly, until autumn, when I again started East on a lecturing tour, which lasted eight months. During this time I averaged one lecture per day. At times, for the space of an entire week, I did not get as much sleep as I needed in one night, and the work I did in those eight months was enough to break down the strongest and healthiest constitution. I spoke in all the more notable cities and towns of Massachusetts, New Hampshire, and Maine. With regard to my success, I will let the Eastern press speak for me. It is not from any motive of vanity that I insert the following notices of the papers, but from a wish to establish in the minds of my readers the fact that my labor was earnest, and not without good results. These extracts are not given in the order in which they appeared; I insert them, taken at random, from hundreds of a similar character. The first is from the Boston Daily Advertiser:

"Mr. Luther Benson, of Indiana, delivered a temperance lecture last evening in Faneuil Hall, before a large and enthusiastic audience. * * *

"The meeting was opened with prayer by the Rev. Mr. Cooke, of the Hanover Street Bethel, after which, Mr. E.H. Sheafe introduced the lecturer. The temperance theme is so old and long discussed that it seemed well-nigh impossible to present its merits in a new and attractive way, but Mr. Benson in a simple, straightforward manner, in language clothed with the peculiar western freedom of speech, together with an accent of marked broadness, held the undivided attention of his audience from the beginning of his lecture to the close. The several stories told by the speaker seemed to exactly suit the temper of his hearers, as the frequent applause testified, and altogether it was probably one of the most satisfactory temperance lectures ever delivered in this city. Mr. Benson, who is a reformed drunkard, describes his trials and struggles in overcoming the evils of intemperance in a very impressive manner, awakening a strong interest for the cause which he pleads.

"During his lecture Mr. Benson paid a marked compliment to the old hall in which he was speaking, and the liberty of speech allowed within its portals. Total Abstinence was the one thing needed throughout the land. There could be no such thing as moderate drinking. Prohibition should be enforced, and great results would necessarily follow."

From the Boston Daily Evening Traveler I clip this concerning my lecture at Chelsea:

"Hawthorn Hall was crowded to the very gallery last evening with an audience assembled to listen to a lecture on temperance by Luther Benson, Esq., of Indiana. Mr. Benson is one of the most powerful and eloquent orators that have ever stood before an audience. For one hour and a half he held his audience by a spell. He painted one beautiful picture after another, and each in the very gems of the English language. He was many times interrupted by loud bursts of applause. Words drop from his lips in strains of such impassioned eloquence that they go directly to the hearts of the audience, and his actions are so well suited to his words that you can not remember a gesture. You try in vain to recall the inflection of the voice that moved you to smiles or tears, at the speaker's will. Mr. Benson is a young man and has only been in the lecture field a little over one year; yet at one leap he has taken the very front rank, and is already measuring strength with the oldest and ablest lecturers in the country."

The next is from the Boston Daily Herald:

"TEMPERANCE AT FANEUIL HALL.

"The old cradle of liberty was filled last evening by a large and appreciative audience, assembled to hear Luther Benson, a well-known temperance advocate from Indiana. Mr. E.H. Sheafe, under whose auspices the lecture was held, presided, and the platform was occupied by the Rev. Mr. Cook, who offered prayer, and by Messrs. Timothy Bigelow, Esq., F.S. Harding, Charles West, John Tobias, S.C. Knight, and other well-known temperance workers in this city. Mr. Benson is a reformed man, and, speaking as he did from a terrible experience, he made an excellent impression, and proved himself an orator of tact, talent and ability. A number of his passages were marked with true eloquence and pathos, and for an hour and a quarter he held the closest attention of his large audience in a manner that could only be done by those who are earnest in the cause, and appeal directly to their hearers."

From the Dover (N.H.) Democrat, this:

"Luther Benson, Esq., spoke to the largest audience ever gathered in the City Hall, last night. Notwithstanding the snow, more than fourteen hundred people crowded themselves in the hall, while hundreds went away for want of even standing-room. He has created a perfect storm of enthusiasm for himself in the cause he so earnestly and eloquently advocates. Last night was Mr. Benson's fourth speech in this city, each one delivered without notes or manuscript, and with no repetition. He goes from here to Great Falls and Berwick. Next Sunday he returns to this city, and speaks here for the last time in City Hall at half past seven o'clock. There never has been a lecturer among us that could repeatedly draw increased audiences, and certainly no man - not even Gough - ever so stirred all classes of our people on the subject of temperance as has Benson. The receipts at the door last evening were about one hundred and forty dollars. A number who had purchased tickets previous to the lecture were unable to get in the hall."

And this from the Pittsburg (Pa.) Gazette:

"Luther Benson, Esq., of Indiana, has just closed one of the most powerful temperance lectures ever delivered here. The house was one solid mass of people, with not one spare inch of standing-room. For nearly two hours he held the audience as by magic. At the close a large number signed the pledge, some of them the hardest drinkers here. The people are so delighted with his good work that they have secured him for another lecture Wednesday evening."

The next extract is from the Manchester (N.H.) Press:

"Smyth's Hall was completely filled, seats and standing room, at two o'clock Sunday afternoon, with an audience which came to hear Luther Benson. The officers of the Reform Club, clergymen and reformed drunkards occupied seats upon the platform. Mr. Benson is a native of Indiana, and says he has been a drunkard from six years of age. He was within three months of graduation from college when he was expelled for drunkenness. Then he studied for a lawyer, and was admitted to practice, being drunk while studying, and drunk while engaged in a case. At length he reduced himself to poverty, pawning all he had for drink. At length he started to reform, and though he had once fallen, he was determined to persevere. Since his reformation two years ago he had been giving temperance lectures. He is a young man, a powerful, swinging sort of speaker, with a good command of language, original, with peculiar intonation, pronunciation and idioms, sometimes rough, but eminently popular with his audiences. He spoke for an hour and a half steadily, wiping the perspiration from his face at intervals, taking up the greater part of his address with his personal experience. He said he had had delirium tremens several times, once for fifteen days, and gave an exceedingly minute and graphic description of his torments. A number of men signed the pledge at the close of the meeting, Among them was one man, who sat in front of the audience and kept drinking from a bottle he had, evidently in a spirit of bravado, but at the conclusion of the address he signed the pledge, crying like a child."

From the Saltsburg Press, of Pennsylvania, I copy the following:

"On Monday evening, 29th inst., the people of our staid and quiet little town had their dormant spirits stirred to their inmost depths, by an eloquent and thrilling lecture delivered in the Presbyterian church by Luther Benson, Esq., a native of Indianapolis, Indiana, who chose for his topic "Total Abstinence." He opened his lecture by delineating in the most touching and beautiful language the almost heavenly happiness resulting in a total abstinence from all intoxicating beverages, and by his well-aimed contrasts demonstrated that, in the use of those beverages, even in a temperate degree, there was but one result - drunkenness and eternal death. He was no advocate of temperance; that is, the temperate use of anything hurtful. Did not believe that anything vicious could be tampered with, without harm coming from it. He argued to a final and satisfactory conclusion, that in the use of alcoholic beverages there could be no such thing as temperance; that the man who took a drink now and then would make it convenient to take more drinks now than he would then, and in the end would as surely fill a drunkard's grave as the man who persistently abused the beverage in its use. His description of the two paths through life was a most beautiful word picture. That of sobriety leading through bright green fields, over flowery plains, by pleasant rivulets, where all was peace and harmony, and over which the spirit of heaven itself seemed to brood and watch; and that of drunkenness, in which all the miseries and tortures of the imaginary hell were concentrated in a living death; of blighted hopes, of wasted life, of ruined homes, of broken hearts, of a conscience goaded to an insanity - to a madness - to fairly wallow in the Lethean draft, that memory might be robbed of its poignant goadings; that the poor, helpless, and degraded victim might escape its horrors in oblivion.

"He had been a victim in the toils of the monster for fifteen years; had endured all the horrors it inflicted upon its votaries during that time, and made an eloquent appeal to the young men present to choose the right way and walk therein. He pictured the inevitable result in new and convincing arguments holding up his own almost hopeless case as a warning. His description of delirium tremens, while it was frightful, was not overdrawn. He told the simple truth, as any one who has passed through the horrible ordeal can testify.

"We have not space to follow Mr. Benson through his lecture, which was truly original in language, style and delivery. He is a lawyer by profession, about twenty-eight years, and is wonderfully gifted with a pleasing way, rapidly flowing and eloquent language, that carries to the audience the conviction that he is in earnest in the work of total abstinence; that in the effort to reclaim himself he will leave nothing undone to save those who may have started out in life impressed with the belief that there is pleasure and enjoyment under the influence of intoxication. That he will accomplish good there is no doubt. He goes into the work under the influence of the Holy Spirit; maintaining that the grace of God alone can work a thorough reformation. We have heard Gough lecture, but maintain that the eloquent, forcible, humorous, pathetic, and convincing language of Mr. Benson is of a better and higher order, and will prove more effectual in touching the hearts of those who stand upon the verge of ruin.

"Mr. Benson will lecture this (Tuesday) evening, in the Presbyterian church. Doors open at 6:30; lecture commencing at 7:30. The lecture this evening will be on a different subject, and no part of the lecture of last evening will be repeated.

"As a result of the lecture Monday evening, one hundred and sixty-two persons signed the pledge."

With reference to the lecture delivered at Faneuil Hall, the Boston Temperance Album gives the succeeding synopsis:

"Mr. Benson, on being introduced, paid the following eloquent tribute to the Hall:

"Ladies and gentlemen: It is with emotions such as I have never experienced upon any former occasion, that I stand before you to-night in this, the birthplace of American liberty. It was in this hall that was first inaugurated the grand march of revolution and liberty that has gilded the page of the history of our time with the most glorious achievements of the patriot that the world has ever had to admire. It was here that was inaugurated those immortal principles that caused revolution to rise in fire, and go down in freedom, amid the ruins and relics of oppression. It was here that the beacon of liberty first blazed, and the rainbow of freedom rose on the cloud of war; and as a result, of the patriotism and heroism of our fore-fathers, liberty has erected her altars here in the very garden of the globe, and the genius of the earth worship at her feet. And here in this garden of the West, here in this land of aspiring hope, where innocence is equity, and talent is triumph, the exile from every land finds a home where his youth may be crowned with happiness, and the sun of life's evening go down with the unmolested hope of a glorious immortality. Who is not proud of being an American citizen, and walking erect and secure under the Stars and Stripes?

"If there be a place on earth where the human mind, unfettered by tyrannical institutions, may rise to the summit of intellectual grandeur, it is here. If there be a country where the human heart, in public and in private, may burst forth in unrestrained adulation to the God that made it, it is here, where the immortal heroes and patriots of more than one hundred years ago succeeded in establishing these United States, as the 'land of the free and the home of the brave.' Here, then, human excellence must attain to the summit of its glory. Mind constitutes the majesty of man, virtue his true nobility. The tide of improvement which is now flowing like another Niagara through the land, is destined to flow on down to the latest posterity, and it will bear on its mighty bosom our virtues, or our vices, our glory, or our shame, or whatever else we may transmit as an inheritance. Thus it depends upon ourselves whether the moth of immortality and the vampire of luxury shall prove the overthrow of this country, or whether knowledge and virtue, like pillars, shall support her against the whirlwinds of war, ambition, corruption, and the remorseless tooth of time. And while assembled here to-night, in this, the very cradle of liberty, let us not forget that there are evils to be shunned and avoided by us as individuals and as a common people.

"It is about one of these evils that is threatening the stability, prosperity, and happiness of this whole country that I would talk to you to-night. Let us approach near to each other and talk, if possible, soul to soul, and heart to heart, I would talk to you to-night of liberty, that liberty that frees us, body, soul, and spirit, from the slavery of the intoxicating bowl; a slavery more soul-wearing and life-destroying than any Egyptian bondage. Why, it is but a few years ago that this whole continent rocked to its very center on the question as to whether human slavery should endure upon its soil! That was but the slavery of the body, a slavery for this life; and that was bad enough, but the slavery about which I talk to you is a slavery not only of the body, but of the soul, and of the spirit; a slavery not only for this life, but a slavery that goes beyond the gates of the tomb, and reaches out into an infinite eternity. The slavery of intoxication, unlike human slavery, is confined to no particular section, climate, or society; for it wars on all mankind. It has for its home this whole world. It has the flesh for its mother and the devil for its father. It stands out a headless, heartless, eyeless, earless, soulless monster of gigantic and fabulous proportions."

As a *very few* persons have said my labors in the cause of Temperance were not, and are not, productive of good, I will give just very short extracts from a number of letters which I have received from persons who ought to know:

FRANKFORT, IND., October 18, 1875.

LUTHER BENSON, ESQ. - _My Dear Sir_ - Yours of the 14th is before me for answer, and, although very busily engaged in court, I can not refrain from answering at some length. First, I will say, "I have kept the faith." Though "the fight" is not yet over, my emancipation from the terrible thralldom is measurably complete. Occasional twinges of appetite yet admonish me to maintain my vigilance. It was while struggling with one of these that your letter came like a messenger from heaven to encourage and strengthen me. Not a day passes but that I think of you, and to your wise counsel and affectionate admonition, under Providence, I owe my beginning and continuance in this well-doing. * * * May the Lord spare you to "open the lips of truth" to those who, like myself, will perish without a revelation of their danger. With high esteem and sincere affection, I am, ever your friend,

SALEM, MASS., October 29, 1875.

BRO. BENSON - I write you these few lines to cheer your heart, and assure you that your labor in Salem has not been in vain in the Lord's cause (the Temperance Reform). Our friend and brother,  -, from Beverly, was over at our meeting on Wednesday evening last, and it would do your heart good to see the change in him. He will never forget Luther Benson, for it was your first speech in Salem that saved him. -

I desire now to come down to the very near present, as some claim that my late *afflictions* and sore misfortunes have extinguished my capacity for good:

MEMPHIS, MO., Feb. 14, 1878.

DEAR BENSON - I know of my personal knowledge that you did a grand work here. Bro. B., you remember my pointing out to you a Dr.  -, and telling you what a persecutor of churches he was, and how hard he drank. He in two nights after you were here signed the pledge, and in telling his experience, said that you saved him - that no other person had ever been able to impress him as you did.

   Truly, -


- , Jan. 1, 1878.

 MY VERY DEAR FRIEND - I wish I could be with you and knee with you as in the past, and hear your faith in God. Here is my hand forever. You have done more for me than all the shepherds on the bleak hillsides of this black world.

   Lovingly,  -

TERRE HAUTE, IND., Feb. 22, 1878.

DEAR BENSON - You have done more for me than all the men and women on earth. One year ago I heard you lecture on Temperance in Lafayette. Then I was a poor outcast drunkard; you saved me. I am now a sober man and a Christian. -

I could furnish thousands of such testimonials as the above, but deem these sufficient to convince any honest person that my toil is not in vain.

From one of the journals of my native State I clip the concluding extract:

"Luther Benson, the gifted inebriate orator, is still struggling against the demon of strong drink. He spoke at Jeffersonville recently, and in the middle of his discourse became so chagrined and disheartened at his repeated failures at reform, that he took his seat and burst into a flood of tears. He has since connected himself with the church, and has professed religion. May his new resolves and associations strengthen him in the line of duty. But, like the man among the tombs, the demons of appetite have taken full possession of his soul, and riot in every vein and fiber of his being. It is a fearful thraldom to be encompassed with the wild hallucinations begotten through a life of dissipation and debauchery. The strongest resolves at reform are broken as ropes of sand. All the moral faculties are made tributary to the one ruling passion - drink, drink, drink! But still his repeated resolves and heroic efforts betoken a greatness of soul rarely witnessed. May he yet live to see the devils that so sorely beset him running furiously down a steep place into the sea, and sink forever from his annoyance. But when they do come out of the man, instead of entering a herd of heedless swine for their coursers to the deep, may they ride, booted and spurred, every saloon-keeper who has contributed to make Luther Benson what he is, to the very verge of despair, and to the brink of hell's yawning abyss."

I might give many more well written and flattering criticisms, but from the foregoing the reader can determine in what estimation to hold my labor. For myself I am not solicitous for anything beyond escape from my thraldom, and that peace which is the sure accompaniment of a temperate Christian life. If I thought that my readers were of the opinion held by some of my enemies that my lectures have not been productive of good, I could quote from numberless private letters received from all parts of the land, in which I am assured of the good results which have crowned my humble efforts - in which I am told of very many instances where my words of entreaty and self-humiliation have been the means of bringing back from the darkness and death of intemperance, fathers, husbands, sons, and brothers who were on the road to destruction. I have letters from the wives, mothers, and sisters of these men, invoking the blessings of heaven upon me for the peace and happiness thus restored to them. I have letters from little children thanking me also for giving them back their fathers, and I thank God from the depths of my torn and desolate heart that I have been the humble instrument of good in these cases. In my darkest hours, when I feel that all is lost, when hope seems to soar away from me to the far-off heavens from which she first descended to this world, these letters, which I often read, and over which I have so often wept grateful tears, give me strength and courage to face the struggle before me. My most earnest prayer to God has been that I may do some good to compensate in some measure for the talent which he gave me, and which I have so sadly wasted. I have avoided mentioning the names of the many dear friends who have not forsaken me in this last extremity. As I write, name after name, dear to memory, crowds into my mind. I can hardly refrain from giving them a place on these pages, but to mention a few would be manifestly unjust to the remainder, and it is out of my power to print all of them in the space which could be afforded in this small book. But I wish to assure every man and woman who has ever given me a kind word of encouragement, or even a kind look, that they are not and never will be forgotten. Whatever my future fate may be, you did your duty, and God will bless you. Your names are all sacred to me.

# CHAPTER XIV

*At home again - Overwork - Shattered nerves - Downward to hell - Conceive the idea of traveling with some one - Leave Indianapolis on a third tour east in company with Gen. Macauley - Separate from him at Buffalo - I go on to New York alone - Trading clothes for whisky - Delirious wanderings - Jersey City - In the calaboose - Deathly sick - An insane neighbor - Another - In court - "John Dalton" - "Here! your honor" - Discharged - Boston - Drunk - At the residence of Junius Brutus Booth - Lecturing again - Home - Converted - Go to Boston - Attend the Moody and Sankey meetings - Get drunk - Home once more - Committed to the asylum - Reflections - The shadow which whispered - "Go away!"*

I returned home from this second tour in the Eastern States in April, 1876, with shattered nerves and weary brain, but instead of resting, I went on lecturing until my overworked mind and body could no longer hold out, and then it was, after nearly two years of sobriety, that I once more fell. For weeks before this disaster overtook me, I was actually an irresponsible maniac. My pulse was never lower than one hundred to the minute, and much of the time it ran up to one hundred and twenty. I was so weak that with all my energy aroused I could only move about with feeble steps, and a constant anxiety and longing for something to drink preyed upon me. I was not content to remain in one place, but wanted to be going somewhere all the time, I cared not where. In this condition I dragged along my existence for weeks, until at last, driven to a frenzy, reason fled, and I plunged headlong into the horrors of

Luther Benson

another debauch. My downward course appeared to be accelerated by the very struggles which I had made to rise during the past two years. The moment I recovered from one horrible spell another more fierce seized me and plunged me into the very depths of hell. I now conceived the idea of getting some one to travel with me, thinking that by this means I could perhaps throw off the morbid gloom and melancholy which hung over me. But again I did the very thing I should not have done - I lectured.

On the 30th of September, 1876, I started from Indianapolis, in company with Gen. Dan. Macauley, on a third lecturing tour East. I was drunk when we started, and remained in that accursed state during the journey. At Buffalo, New York, we got separated, thence I went to New York city alone, where I continued drinking until I had no money. I then commenced to pawn my clothes - first, my vest; second, a pair of new boots, worth fourteen dollars; I got a quart of whisky, an old and worn-out pair of shoes, and ten cents in money, for my boots. I drank up the whisky, and traded off my overcoat. It was worth sixty dollars. I realized about five cents on the dollar, and all the horrors of all hells ever heard of, for I was attacked with the delirium tremens. By some means, of which I am entirely ignorant, I got across the river, into Jersey City, and was there arrested and lodged in the calaboose, in which I remained from Saturday until the following Monday. I suffered more in the forty-eight hours embraced in that time than I ever before or since suffered in the same length of time. I do not know the hour, but it was getting dark on that Saturday evening, when I got deathly sick, and commenced vomiting. I continued vomiting until Monday. Nothing that I swallowed would remain on my stomach. About eight o'clock Saturday evening the authorities, the police officers, put a large number of men and boys, who were arrested for being drunk, in the room in which I was confined. By midnight there were fourteen of us in a small, poorly-ventilated, dirty room. Planks extended around the room on three sides, and on these those who could get a place lay down. Among the number of "drunks" imprisoned with me were some of the worst and largest roughs of Jersey City, and these inhuman wretches, in the absence of the police, threatened; to take my life if I vomited again. In the room adjoining ours a madman was confined, and I don't think he ceased kicking and screaming a moment from Saturday night until Monday. In the room just across the narrow hall, fronting ours, was an insane woman, who swore she had two souls, one of which was in hell! She, too, kept up an incessant, piteous wailing, begging some one, ever and anon, with piercing screams, to bring back her lost soul! Indianapolis is more civilized than Jersey City in respect to her prisons, but not with respect to her police. And I am pretty sure that, as managed by its present superintendent, the unfortunate insane are in no other State cared for as they are in the Indiana asylum, and in no other State is the appropriation for running such a noble institution so beggarly as in ours. I have visited other asylums, and am now an inmate of this, and I know whereof I speak.

The reader may have a faint idea of my sufferings while in the Jersey City calaboose when I tell him that the least noise pierced my brain like a knife. I can in fancy and in my dreams hear the wild screams of that woman yet. On Monday morning we were marched together to a room, and I saw that there were about fifty persons all told under arrest. Among the number were many women, and I write with sorrow that their language was more profane and indecent than that of the men. I stood as in a nightmare and heard the judge say from time to time - "Five dollars" - "Ten dollars" - "Ten days" - "Fifteen days" - and so on. I was so weak that I found it almost out of my power to stand up, and as the various sentences were pronounced my heart gave a quick throb of agony. I felt that a sentence of ten days would kill me. At this moment "John Dalton" was called. I answered "Here, your Honor!" for Dalton was the name I had assumed. My offense was read - and the officer who arrested me volunteered the statement that I was not disorderly, and that I had not been creating any disturbance. I felt called upon to plead my own case before the judge, and without waiting for his permission I began to speak. It was life or death with me, and for ten minutes I spoke as I never spoke before and have never spoken since. I pierced through his judicial armor and touched his pity, else the fear of being talked to death influenced him, to discharge me with the generous advice to leave the city. Either way I was free, and was not long in getting across the river into New York, where I succeeded in finding General Macauley who saw that my toilet was once more arranged in a respectable manner. That night we started for Boston, and arrived there on Tuesday morning. I got drunk immediately and remained drunk until Saturday, on which memorable day I went in company with the General to Junius Brutus Booth's residence, at Manchester, Mass., where I staid, well provided for, until I got sober. I then began to fill my engagements, and for six weeks lectured almost every day and night. I again broke down and came home. I finally got sober once more and did not drink anything until in January last, when I again fell. I went to Jeffersonville to lecture, and while there became converted. Had I then ceased to work and given my worn-out body and mind a much needed rest, I would have to-day been standing up before the world a free and happy man. But my desire to see and tell every one of the new joy which I had found controlled me, and for six weeks I spoke every day, and often twice a day. I started east again and went to Boston. I attended the Moody and Sankey meetings, but was troubled with I know not what. All the time an unnatural feeling seemed to have possession of me.

One afternoon, just after getting off my knees from prayer, a strange spell came over me and before I could realize what I was doing, the devil hurried me into a saloon, where I began to drink recklessly, and knew nothing more for two or three days. Then I awoke, I knew not where. Some of my friends found me and sent me home. I now suffered more mental torture than I experienced on sobering up from any other spree I was ever on. I believed firmly that I was saved; that my appetite for liquor was forever gone. I felt now that there was no hope for me. Oh, the despairing days and long black nights of agony unspeakable that followed this debauch! In time I recovered physical health, and began to lecture, though under greater difficulties than ever before. I was so harrassed by my own shame and the world's doubts that within a month I again got drunk. While on this spree my friends made out the necessary papers, and I was committed to the Indiana Hospital for the Insane. Here, then, I am to-day, very near the end of my most wretched and misspent life. How can I tell the emotions which swell in my heart? It is on the record of this asylum that I was brought here June 4th, a victim of intemperance. Everything is being done for me that can be done, but I feel that my case is hopeless unless help comes from above. Ordinarily restraint and proper attention to diet and rest would in time cure aggravated cases of that peculiar insanity which manifests itself in an abnormal and excessive demand for liquor. But with me the spell returns after months of sobriety with a force which I am powerless to resist, as the reader has seen in the several instances given in this autobiography. The rule of treatment for patients here varies with the different characters of the patients. The impressions which I had formed of insane asylums was very different from those which have come from my sojourn among the insane. There is less screaming and violence than I thought there would be, and for most of the time the wards in which the better class of patients are confined are as still and apparently as peaceful as a home circle. The horror experienced during the first week's, or first two weeks' confinement wears off, and one gradually forgets that he is in a house for the mad. Many amusing cases come under my observation, but there are others which excite various feelings of pity, disgust, fear, and horror. There is, for instance, a man in "my ward" who imagines that he has murdered all his relations. Another believes that he swallowed and carries within him a living mule which compels him to walk on his hands as well as his feet. One poor fellow can not be convinced but assassins are hourly trying to stab or shoot him. One is afraid to eat for fear of being poisoned, and another wants to disembowel himself. Twice a day the wards, which number from thirty to forty patients under the charge of two attendants, one or the other of whom is constantly on duty, are taken out for a walk in the beautiful grounds around the asylum. Sometimes, when it is thought that the patient will be benefited, and when he is really well but still not in a condition to be discharged, he is allowed the freedom of the grounds. After I had been here two weeks I was permitted to go out on the grounds alone. But my feelings are about the same outside the building as inside. Even as I write I feel that there is a devil within me which is demanding me to go away from this place. I want whisky, and would at this moment barter my soul for a pint of the hellish poison. I have now been here a little over a month. Like all the other patients, I am kindly treated. Our beds are clean, and our food is well prepared, such as it is, and it is really much better than could be expected on the appropriation made by the last Legislature. I doubt if there is another institution of the kind in the United States that can be compared with this in the ability, justice, kindness, and noble and unswerving honesty of its management. Dr. Everts, the superintendent, is a gentleman whom I have not the honor to know personally, but whose commanding intelligence, and equally great heart, are venerated by all who do know him.

This is the fourth day of July, and I have written to my friends to come and take me away - for what purpose I dare not think. I am utterly desolate and miserable, and dare not look forward to the future, for I dread to face the uncertain and unknown TO-COME. To stay here is worse than madness, in my present condition, and to go away may be death. O, that some power higher than earth would reach forth a hand and save me from myself! I can not remain here without abusing the kindness and trust of a great institution, nor can I go away, I fear, without bringing disgrace on my friends, and shame and death on myself. God of mercy, help me! I know how useless it would be to lock me up in solitary confinement, and I think my attendant physician also feels that I can not be saved by any means within the reach of the asylum. With others not insane, but cursed with that insanity for drink which, if not checked, will soon or late lead to the destruction of reason and life itself, there is a chance to restore them from the curse to a life of honor and usefulness, and no means should be left untried which may ultimately save them, especially the young who, but for this curse infernal, might rise to a useful and even august manhood.

The shadows of the evening are settling upon the face of the earth. Now and then the report of a cannon in the direction of the city recalls what day it is, and I am reminded that crowds are thronging the streets for the purpose of witnessing the display of holiday fireworks; but vain to me such mimicry. A tall and mysterious shadow, more dark and awful than any which will steal among the graves of the old churchyard to-night, has risen and now stands beside whispering in the stillness - "Go away!"

# CHAPTER XV

*A sleepless night - Try to write on the following day but fail - My friends consult with the officers of the institution - I am discharged - Go to Indianapolis and get drunk - My wanderings and horrible sufferings - Alcohol - The tyrant whom all should slay - What is lost by the drunkard - Is anything gained by the use of liquor? - Never touch it in any form - It leads to ruin and death - Better blow your brains out - My condition at present - The end.*

After writing the words "go away," which close the preceding chapter, I lay down and tried to compose my thoughts, but the effort was futile. I passed a sleepless night, and when morning came I had fully resolved to leave the hospital if in my power to do so. During the forenoon I took up my pencil a number of times for the purpose of writing, but I was so disturbed in mind that I could not write a line intelligibly, and I will here say that from that day, July fifth, to this, September fifteenth, the manuscript remained untouched in the hands of a very dear friend, to whom I am under many obligations for his clear advice and judgment on matters of this sort as well as on others. I will now write this, the fifteenth and last chapter of this book; and in order to make the story of my life complete up to this date, I will go back and resume the thread of the narrative where it was left off on the evening of the fourth of July. It will be remembered that in my last chapter I spoke of having written letters to some of my friends desiring them to come and ask for my discharge. I awaited impatiently their coming, but when they came, which was on the sixth of July, I think, they were undecided whether it would be better for me to "go away," or remain longer at the asylum, but I plead to go, as if my life depended upon it. After consultation with the authorities at the hospital, who were clearly of the opinion that they had no right to detain me under the circumstances, and who, therefore, felt it incumbent upon them to discharge me, particularly if my friends were willing, it was by all parties decided that I should go. I felt glad in my heart that the institution was relieved of all responsibility in my case, for I did not wish to bring reproach upon anyone, and I feared if I remained longer I might take some rash step (abusing the generous kindness of my officers) that would do so. They had done their whole duty by me, and it remained for me now to do my duty to myself and friends. But as soon as I got to Indianapolis the pent-up fires of appetite blazed forth, and while on the way to the Union Depot to take the train to Rushville, I gave my friends the slip, and, sneaking like a thief through the alleys, I sought and found an obscure saloon in which I secreted myself and began to drink. I was once more on the road which leads to perdition. The old enemy, who had crawled up the walls of the asylum and slimed himself through my grated windows, and coiled around my heart in frightful dreams, again had me in his possession. Thus began one of the most maniacal and terrible drunks of my life. I became possessed of the wildest and most unreal thoughts that ever entered a crazed brain. I abused and misrepresented my best friends, and cursed everything but the thrice cursed liquor which was burning up my body and soul. I told absurd and terrible stories about the places where I had been, and about the friends who had done most for me. I was insane - as utterly so for the time as the worst case in the asylum. I knew not what I did or said, and yet my actions and words were cunningly contrived to deceive.

For the greater part of the fifteen days which followed I was as unconscious of what I did or said as if I had been dead and buried in the bottom of the sea. What I know of the time I have learned since from the lips of others. The hideous, fiendish serpent of drunkenness possessed my whole being. I felt him in every nerve, bone, sinew, fiber, and drop of blood in my body. There were moments when a glimmer of reason came to me, and with it a pang that shriveled my soul. During the period that I was drinking I was in Rushville, after leaving Indianapolis, Falmouth and Cambridge City. Of course, for the most part of the time, I knew not where I was. As I think of it now, I know that I was in hell. My thirst for whisky was positively maddening. I tried every means to quit, when conscious of my existence: I voluntarily entered the calaboose more than once, and was locked up, but the instant I got out, the madness caused me to fly where liquor was. I drank it in enormous quantities, and smothered without quenching the scorching, blazing fires of hell which were making cinders and ashes of every hope and energy of my being. I made my bed among serpents; I fed on flames and poison; I walked with demons and ghouls; all unutterable and slimy monsters crawled around and over me; every breath that I drew reeked with the odor of death; every beat of my fast-throbbing heart sent the hissing, boiling blood through my veins, which returned and froze about it. I have neither words nor images sufficiently horrible to typify my condition. I became, for the time an abhorred object; the sex of my sainted mother made a wide sweep to pass me by, and dear, little, innocent children fled from me as from a monster. My soul was no longer my own. The fiend Appetite had given it over, bound and helpless, to the fiend Alcohol. I turned by bleared vision towards the vaulted skies, and cursed them because they did not rain fire and brimstone down upon me and destroy me. And yet, oh! how I dreaded to die! The grave opened before me, and a million horrors were in its hollow and black chasm. The scalding tears I shed gave me no relief; the cries I uttered were unheard; and every ear was deaf to my pleadings. At times I thought of the asylum, and I would have given worlds could I have retraced my steps, and slept once more securely within its merciful and protecting walls. O, God! I screamed, why did I leave it? As day after day dragged its endless length along, and no relief came, my despair was a delirium of wretchedness. The sun appeared to be extinguished, and the universe was a void of black, impenetrable darkness, out of which, before and after me, rose the hideous specters, Death and Annihilation. The unimaginable horrors of the tremens were upon me.

Once more hear my voice, you who read! Lose no opportunity to strike a blow at intemperance. It may smile in the rosy face of youth, but do not be deceived; there are agonies unspeakable hidden beneath that smile. Look not on the wine cup when it is red, no matter if the jeweled hand of a princess hold it between you and the light. It is the beginning whose end is degradation, remorse, misery and death! Turn from a glass of beer as from a goblet of reeking and poisoned blood. It is a danger to be shunned. Beware that you do not learn this too late.

Alcohol, ruin, and death go hand in hand. The region over which Alcohol is king is one of decay. It is full of graves. The ghosts of the million joys, he has slain wail amid its ghastly desolations; there are sounds of sobbing orphans there; echoes of widows' shrieks; and the lamentations of fond mothers and wives, heart-broken, vex the realm; youth and age lie here dishonored together; in vain the sweetheart begs her lover to return from its fatal mists; in vain the pure sister calls with trembling tongue for her erring brother. He will not come back. He is the slave of a tyrant who has no compassion and knows no mercy. Oppose this tyrant, all ye who love the home circle better than the bawdy house; fight him all ye who set honor above dishonor; curse him all ye who prefer peace to discord, and law to anarchy; war against him in all ways unceasingly all ye to whom the thought of liberty and safety is dear, to whom happiness and truth are more desirable than misery and falsehood.

What, let me ask, is to be gained by drinking? What blessing comes from forming or indulging the habit? Pause here and think well before you answer. You could not afford to drink if the wealth of a nation were yours, because no man can afford to lose health and happiness if he hopes enjoyment in life. If you are strong, alcohol will destroy your nerves and sap your vigor. If you are weak, it will enfeeble you the more. If you are unhappy, it will only add to your unhappiness. Look at the subject as you will, you can not afford to drink intoxicating liquors. The moment you begin to form the habit of drinking that moment you begin to endanger your reputation, health and happiness, and that of your family and friends also. And let me say right now that you begin to form the habit when you touch your lips to any sort of intoxicating drink the first time. I have drank the sparkle and foam, and the gall and wormwood of all liquors. Do you envy me the horrors through which I have passed? You know how to avoid them. Never touch liquor. If you are bent on going to hell and destruction, choose a nearer and more honorable way by blowing your brains out at once.

A few words more, dear readers, and I will bid you good by. Many of you have no doubt heard of my restored peace and lasting favor with God at Fowler, Indiana. With regard to it and my condition at the present time, I will incorporate in substance the letter which I recently published in reply to inquiries addressed to me from all parts of the country, shortly after that event. I will give the letter with but little change, even at the risk of repeating what is elsewhere recorded. It is as follows:

On the evening of January twenty-first, 1877, at Jeffersonville, Indiana, God pardoned my sins and made me a new creature. For weeks happiness and joy were mine. The appetite - rather my passion - for liquor, which made the present a misery and the future a darkness, was no longer present. Its heavy burdens had fallen from me. Of this there could be no doubt; but I had been educated to believe that "once in grace always in grace," and this led to a fatal deception, a belief that I could not fall; that after God had once pardoned my sins I was as surely saved as if already in Paradise. That they were pardoned I had not a doubt, for the manifestations were as clear as light. Falsely thinking that I was pardoned for all time, my soul grew self-reliant: I became at the same time careless of my religious duties. I neglected to pray, to beware of temptation, and, naturally enough, soon found myself drifting into the society of those who neither loved nor feared God. Had I trusted alone in God and permitted the Savior to lead and keep me, I should not have fallen. Instead, I went back to the world, gave no thanks to God for his mercy and love, and thus dishonoring him, his face was hidden from me.

I went to Boston to speak in Moody and Sankey's meeting. I never once hoped by so doing to be the means of others' salvation; my sole thought was self and selfish ambition. Instead of talking at the Moody meeting, I took a drink of liquor, soon got drunk, and so remained for days. When I came out of the oblivion of that debauch, the agony experienced was terrible. All the shames, all the burning regrets, all the stinging compunctions of conscience I had known on coming out of such debauches before my conversion were almost as joy compared with the misery which preyed upon my heart then. I can not describe the hopeless feeling of remorse which came over me. I lived and moved in a night of misery and no star was in its sky. In the course of a few days I recovered physically so far as to be able to lecture. I prayed in secret, long and often, for a return of that peace which comes from God alone, but in vain. I was justly self-punished. At the end of four or five weeks I fell again, and this time my degradation was deeper than before. I would at times console myself with the thought that my suffering had reached the limit of endurance, and at such times new and still keener agonies would rise in my heart, like harpies, to tear me to atoms.

It was at this time that I was committed to the Hospital for the Insane at Indianapolis. The reader is aware of what took place on my arrival at Indianapolis, after leaving the hospital. I felt somehow that it was my last spree. I kept it up until nature could endure no more. I felt that my stomach was burned up, and that my brain was scalded. I was crucified from my head to the soles of my feet. I began to feel sure that this time I would die, and, when dead, go to the hell which seemed to be open to receive me. July twenty-first I left Indianapolis, and went to Fowler, Indiana, at which place, for five days and nights, I suffered every mental and physical pang that can afflict mortal man. Day and night I prayed God to be merciful, but no relief came. The dark hopelessness in which I lay I can not describe. I felt that I was undeserving of God's pardon or mercy. I had wronged myself, and my friends more than myself; I had trampled upon the love of Christ; I had loved myself amiss and lost myself. The Christian people of Fowler prayed for me; they called a prayer-meeting especially for me, to ask God to have mercy on and save me. On Wednesday night I went to the regular prayer-meeting, and, with a breaking heart, begged, on bended knee, that God would take compassion on me. The next day, July twenty-sixth, was the most wretched day I ever passed on earth. It seemed that whichsoever way I turned, hell's fiercest fires lapped up around my feet. There seemed no escape for me. Like that scorpion girt with flames, flee in any direction I would, I found the misery and suffering increasing. I resolved to commit suicide, but when just in the act of taking my life the Spirit of God restrained me. I met the Rev. Frank Taylor, the pastor at Fowler. I told him my hopeless condition. He cheered me in every way possible. In the evening we took a walk, and it was during this walk, while in the act of reaching my hand down to my pocket to get a chew of tobacco, that I felt a power hold back my hand, and, plainer than any spoken words, this same power told me not to touch it. I obeyed, withdrew my hand, and at that instant the glory of God filled my heart, suffering fled from me, and in its stead came sweet peace.

I had been using enormous quantities of tobacco, and the use of this narcotic increased, if it did not aid in bringing on my appetite for liquor. I have at times suffered keenly from suddenly renouncing its use, but from the time God fully restored me I have not tasted nor touched tobacco and whisky or any other stimulants. Do not understand me as saying that the appetite for them is dead, or that I have had no hours of depression and struggle in which the old Satan tempted me. I expect all my life to wage a battle against him, and to know what sorrow is and pain. But by the grace of God I will dare to do right, and with his help I mean to be victorious in every fight against sin. I will abase myself with a trusting heart, and shrink from all self-esteem at war with the true principles to which a follower of Christ should cling. I will grind myself to dust if by so doing I may have God's grace. I fully realize that left to myself I am nothing. Jesus is not only my Savior; he shall be my guide in all things. His precious blood has redeemed me, and I am at rest in the shadow of the Rifted Rock. Peace dwells within me, and joy and praise to the Father of all mercies fill my soul. To that Father Almighty be the praise. I earnestly desire the prayers of all Christian men and women. Every time you pray ask God to keep and save me with a salvation which shall be everlasting.

# Choose from Thousands of 1stWorldLibrary Classics By

A. M. Barnard
Ada Leverson
Adolphus William Ward
Aesop
Agatha Christie
Alexander Aaronsohn
Alexander Kielland
Alexandre Dumas
Alfred Gatty
Alfred Ollivant
Alice Duer Miller
Alice Turner Curtis
Alice Dunbar
Ambrose Bierce
Amelia E. Barr
Amory H. Bradford
Andrew Lang
Andrew McFarland Davis
Andy Adams
Anna Sewell
Annie Besant
Annie Hamilton Donnell
Annie Payson Call
Annonaymous
Anton Chekhov
Arnold Bennett
Arthur Conan Doyle
Arthur M. Winfield
Arthur Ransome
Atticus
B.H. Baden-Powell
B. M. Bower
Baroness Emmuska Orczy
Baroness Orczy
Basil King
Bayard Taylor
Ben Macomber
Bertha Muzzy Bower
Bjornstjerne Bjornson
Booth Tarkington
Boyd Cable
Bram Stoker
C. Collodi
C. E. Orr
C. M. Ingleby
Carolyn Wells
Catherine Parr Traill
Charles A. Eastman
Charles Dickens

Charles Dudley Warner
Charles Farrar Browne
Charles Ives
Charles Kingsley
Charles Klein
Charles Amory Beach
Charles Hanson Towne
Charles Lathrop Pack
Charles Whibley
Charles Willing Beale
Charlotte M. Braeme
Charlotte M. Yonge
Charlotte Perkins Stetson
Clair W. Hayes
Clarence Day Jr.
Clarence E. Mulford
Clemence Housman
Confucius
Cornelis DeWitt Wilcox
Cyril Burleigh
D. H. Lawrence
Daniel Defoe
David Garnett
Dinah Craik
Don Carlos Janes
Donald Keyhoe
Dorothy Kilner
Dougan Clark
Douglas Fairbanks
E. Nesbit
E.P.Roe
E. Phillips Oppenheim
Earl Barnes
Edgar Rice Burroughs
Edith Van Dyne
Edith Wharton
Edward J. O'Biren
Edward S. Ellis
Edwin L. Arnold
Eleanor Atkins
Eliot Gregory
Elizabeth Gaskell
Elizabeth McCracken
Elizabeth Von Arnim
Ellem Key
Emerson Hough
Emilie F. Carlen
Emily Dickinson
Enid Bagnold

Enilor Macartney Lane
Erasmus W. Jones
Ernie Howard Pie
Ethel Turner
Ethel Watts Mumford
Eugenie Foa
Eugene Wood
Eustace Hale Ball
Evelyn Everett-green
Everard Cotes
F. H. Cheley
F. J. Cross
Federick Austin Ogg
Ferdinand Ossendowski
Francis Bacon
Francis Darwin
Frances Hodgson Burnett
Frances Parkinson Keyes
Frank Gee Patchin
Frank Harris
Frank Jewett Mather
Frank L. Packard
Frank V. Webster
Frederic Stewart Isham
Frederick Trevor Hill
Frederick Winslow Taylor
Friedrich Kerst
Friedrich Nietzsche
Fyodor Dostoyevsky
G.A. Henty
G.K. Chesterton
Gabrielle E. Jackson
Garrett P. Serviss
Gaston Leroux
George A. Warren
George Ade
Geroge Bernard Shaw
George Durston
George Ebers
George Eliot
George Gissing
George MacDonald
George Meredith
George Orwell
George Sylvester Viereck
George Tucker
George W. Cable
George Wharton James
Gertrude Atherton

| | | |
|---|---|---|
| Grace E. King | J. Henri Fabre | Katherine Stokes |
| Grace Gallatin | J. M. Barrie | L. A. Abbot |
| Grant Allen | J. Macdonald Oxley | L. T. Meade |
| Guillermo A. Sherwell | J. S. Fletcher | L. Frank Baum |
| Gulielma Zollinger | J. S. Knowles | Latta Griswold |
| Gustav Flaubert | J. Storer Clouston | Laura Lee Hope |
| H. A. Cody | Jack London | Laurence Housman |
| H. B. Irving | Jacob Abbott | Lawrence Beasley |
| H.C. Bailey | James Allen | Leo Tolstoy |
| H. G. Wells | James Andrews | Leonid Andreyev |
| H. H. Munro | James Baldwin | Lewis Carroll |
| H. Irving Hancock | James DeMille | Lewis Sperry Chafer |
| H. Rider Haggard | James Joyce | Lilian Bell |
| H. W. C. Davis | James Lane Allen | Lloyd Osbourne |
| Hamilton Wright Mabie | James Lane Allen | Louis Hughes |
| Hans Christian Andersen | James Oliver Curwood | Louis Tracy |
| Harold Avery | James Oppenheim | Louisa May Alcott |
| Harold McGrath | James Otis | Lucy Fitch Perkins |
| Harriet Beecher Stowe | James R. Driscoll | Lucy Maud Montgomery |
| Harry Houidini | Jane Austen | Lydia Miller Middleton |
| Helent Hunt Jackson | Janet Aldridge | Lyndon Orr |
| Helen Nicolay | Jens Peter Jacobsen | M. Corvus |
| Hendrik Conscience | Jerome K. Jerome | M. H. Adams |
| Hendy David Thoreau | John Burroughs | Margaret E. Sangster |
| Henri Barbusse | John Cournos | Margaret Vandercook |
| Henrik Ibsen | John F. Kennedy | Margret Penrose |
| Henry Adams | John Gay | Maria Edgeworth |
| Henry Ford | John Glasworthy | Maria Thompson Daviess |
| Henry Frost | John Habberton | Mariano Azuela |
| Henry James | John Joy Bell | Marion Polk Angellotti |
| Henry Jones Ford | John Kendrick Bangs | Mark Overton |
| Henry Seton Merriman | John Milton | Mark Twain |
| Henry W Longfellow | John Philip Sousa | Mary Austin |
| Herbert A. Giles | Jonas Lauritz Idemil Lie | Mary Catherine Crowley |
| Herbert N. Casson | Jonathan Swift | Mary Cole |
| Herman Hesse | Joseph A. Altsheler | Mary Hastings Bradley |
| Homer | Joseph Carey | Mary Roberts Rinehart |
| Honore De Balzac | Joseph Conrad | Mary Rowlandson |
| Horace Walpole | Joseph E. Badger Jr | M. Wollstonecraft Shelley |
| Horatio Alger Jr. | Joseph Hergesheimer | Maud Lindsay |
| Howard Pyle | Joseph Jacobs | Max Beerbohm |
| Howard R. Garis | Jules Vernes | Myra Kelly |
| Hugh Lofting | Julian Hawthrone | Nathaniel Hawthrone |
| Hugh Walpole | Julie A Lippmann | Nicolo Machiavelli |
| Humphry Ward | Justin Huntly McCarthy | O. F. Walton |
| Ian Maclaren | Kakuzo Okakura | Oscar Wilde |
| Inez Haynes Gillmore | Kenneth Grahame | Owen Johnson |
| Irving Bacheller | Kenneth McGaffey | P.G. Wodehouse |
| Israel Abrahams | Kate Langley Bosher | Paul and Mabel Thorne |
| Ivan Turgenev | Kate Langley Bosher | Paul G. Tomlinson |
| J.G.Austin | Katherine Cecil Thurston | Paul Severing |

Percy Brebner
Peter B. Kyne
Plato
R. Derby Holmes
R. L. Stevenson
R. S. Ball
Rabindranath Tagore
Rahul Alvares
Ralph Bonehill
Ralph Henry Barbour
Ralph Victor
Ralph Waldo Emmerson
Rene Descartes
Rex Beach
Rex E. Beach
Richard Harding Davis
Richard Jefferies
Richard Le Gallienne
Robert Barr
Robert Frost
Robert Gordon Anderson
Robert L. Drake
Robert Lansing
Robert Lynd
Robert Michael Ballantyne
Robert W. Chambers
Rosa Nouchette Carey
Rudyard Kipling
Samuel B. Allison

Samuel Hopkins Adams
Sarah Bernhardt
Sarah C. Hallowell
Selma Lagerlof
Sherwood Anderson
Sigmund Freud
Standish O'Grady
Stanley Weyman
Stella Benson
Stephen Crane
Stewart Edward White
Stijn Streuvels
Swami Abhedananda
Swami Parmananda
T. S. Ackland
T. S. Arthur
The Princess Der Ling
Thomas A. Janvier
Thomas A Kempis
Thomas Anderton
Thomas Bailey Aldrich
Thomas Bulfinch
Thomas De Quincey
Thomas H. Huxley
Thomas Hardy
Thomas More
Thornton W. Burgess
U. S. Grant
Valentine Williams

Various Authors
Vaughan Kester
Victor Appleton
Virginia Woolf
Walter Camp
Walter Scott
Washington Irving
Wilbur Lawton
Wilkie Collins
Willa Cather
Willard F. Baker
William Dean Howells
William le Queux
W. Makepeace Thackeray
William W. Walter
Winston Churchill
Yei Theodora Ozaki
Yogi Ramacharaka
Young E. Allison
Zane Grey

www.ingramcontent.com/pod-product-compliance
Lightning Source LLC
Chambersburg PA
CBHW051837170626
46807CB00003B/1229